Evaluating Voice Therapy

Evaluating Voice Therapy
Measuring the
Effectiveness of Treatment

PAUL CARDING, BA, DIP CCS, MRCSLT, PhD

Senior Lecturer in Voice Pathology, Department of Surgery,
University of Newcastle upon Tyne
Clinical Head, Speech and Voice Therapy Department, Freeman
Hospital, Newcastle upon Tyne

W

WHURR PUBLISHERS
LONDON AND PHILADELPHIA

© 2000 Whurr Publishers
First published 2000 by
Whurr Publishers Ltd
19b Compton Terrace, London N1 2UN, England, and
325 Chestnut Street, Philadelphia PA 19106, USA

British Library Cataloguing in Publication Data
A catalogue record for this book is available from the
British Library.

ISBN 1 86156 162 8

Contents

Foreword

Evaluating Voice Therapy fills a gap in voice literature. Its author, Paul Carding, is the first Senior Lecturer in Speech and Language Pathology in the UK, and is a leading authority on the outcomes of voice therapy. He has a growing international reputation in this field enhanced by the highly successful courses in the Evaluation of Therapy which he organises regularly at the University of Newcastle upon Tyne's Freeman Hospital.

Evaluating Voice Therapy is a timely publication given the current and ongoing interest in evidence-based practice. The volume emphasises the multidimensional requirements of good voice evaluation and represents a key text in voice outcomes applicable to all dysphonic patients.

Any professional whose interventions may effect voice quality will find this an invaluable source book. It will also provide a useful grounding for undergraduates in voice therapy and laryngology.

It has been my great pleasure to work with Paul Carding for the past five years. This volume is a fitting tribute to his knowledge, energy and vision for the future of voice therapy.

Janet A. Wilson
Professor of Otolaryngology,
Head and Neck Surgery,
University of Newcastle upon Tyne

Acknowledgements

I would like to thank Dr Gerry Docherty and Mrs Irmgarde Horsley of the Department of Speech, University of Newcastle upon Tyne, for their contribution to the research which underpins this book.

Dedication

I would like to dedicate this book to my family. My wife, Kate, is a constant source of support and energy to me. My children, Jamie and Jenny, are my inspiration.

Chapter 1
Why do we need evidence of treatment effectiveness?

As speech and language therapists, we know surprisingly little about whether or not our treatments work. Most of our therapeutic techniques have not been properly evaluated. We have a professional responsibility to establish evidence of treatment effectiveness and, if we do not do this, then others will do it for us (Kluppel-Vetter, 1985). Past experience has shown that this may result in misguided, unrepresentative and harmful research evidence (Frattali, 1998). We need to be proactive in designing studies of treatment effectiveness that are scientifically robust and clinically valid.

There are clinical, financial and patient-centred reasons why we need evidence of the effectiveness of treatment.

Clinical reasons

Clinically, we aim to provide the most appropriate treatment to accomplish the best outcome for our patients. To achieve this, the clinician must constantly evaluate his or her own practice and constantly evaluate alternative practice. Clinicians who systematically investigate the nature, quality and outcomes of their treatments are likely to provide high-quality clinical practice.

A clinician who constantly evaluates other intervention options is likely to provide a comprehensive, knowledgeable and eclectic approach to treatment. The clinician is able to compare and contrast treatment programmes with the aim of achieving the best possible outcome for the patient.

Financial reasons

Financially, the profession needs evidence of providing 'value for money'. In an ever-worsening situation of increased demand for limited resources, health-care purchasers have to rationalise their decisions. They wish to

1

maximise the best use of health service money to the largest population possible. Before allocating resources to a treatment they will evaluate the evidence.

> The competitive edge will go to the health care professionals who can demonstrate most effectively – based on hard data – what beneficial outcomes their services can deliver. (Boston, 1994, page 35)

Services with poor evidence of treatment effectiveness are likely to receive limited financial support as a consequence. Milne and Hicks (1996) recognised that the decisions about the finance of service provisions should not be taken entirely on the evidence of effectiveness alone and need to be supplemented with evidence concerning other dimensions of quality. Maxwell (1992) defined six further dimensions of quality, which included accessibility, relevance, equity, acceptability and efficiency. It is true that health care purchasers should not fund services only on their evidence base of effectiveness. However, neither should they continue to purchase accessible, relevant and equitable services that cannot demonstrate that they produce any beneficial effect for the patient.

Patient-centred reasons

There are also patient-centred reasons why we should be concerned with treatment effectiveness. The patient assumes that the clinician has professional integrity and aims to give him or her the best treatment. However, there is also the increasing importance of 'patient power'. Consumers of health services are exerting more and more political pressure and telling us what *they* expect. Whatever health service system we work in, the consumer is, either directly or indirectly, also the purchaser of these services. Today's health service delivery:

> ... has an unprecedented emphasis on meeting the consumer's demands and, consequently, providers are increasingly being held accountable for meeting or even exceeding a variety of consumer expectation. (Rao et al., 1998, page 89)

Why is there so little evidence of treatment effectiveness?

Why is it that our profession currently lacks the evidence to support claims of treatment effectiveness? Boston (1994) lists a number of reasons for the lack of clinical evidence. These include: the lack of a common language for reporting data; a lack of experience or training in data collection for many professional members; no central (professional body) coordination of data; the absence of standardised formats and descriptions of outcomes; no strong networks for data sharing; incompatible software for registering and sharing data; confusions between cause and effect among patients with multiple problems; the complex nature of communication disorders in general; and a history of focusing on process rather than outcome. There is no doubt that these factors represent very real obstacles to treatment evaluation. Most of them are, of course, problems of our own making and are therefore redeemable.

Ellwood (1988) believes that one of the major reasons why there has not been more research into clinical effectiveness has been the vehement attitude of the clinician that 'less paperwork means more patient-care'. There is a perceived reluctance to adopt the principles of outcome measurement because of fear of losing professional control. Iezoni (1994) states that measurement of treatment outcomes requires a degree of vigilance beyond the tolerance of most clinicians. She also suggests that good treatment evidence relies on two vital methodologies: a measure of the outcome itself and a way to account for patient variables in determining outcomes. The first methodology requires good outcome measures, which, in most cases, we do not have. This issue is discussed in Chapter 4. The second method requires experimental control, which may then not reflect clinical reality. This issue is discussed in Chapter 2. The ease with which outcomes of an intervention can be measured will also influence the amount of research undertaken. Hope (1995) gave a good example of this when he compared the relative ease of measuring the outcome for an intervention aimed at correcting an acute medical problem, compared with the less clear-cut, longer-term outcomes of interventions for people with chronic disease, or those requiring complicated multi-dimensional treatment programmes.

Demming (1982) blames the lack of effectiveness data on a historical perspective – where most managers and clinicians have based decisions on clinical hunches instead of evidence-based knowledge. This view was reflected by Sir Michael Peckham, the Director of Research and Development (R&D), when the UK Department of Health launched its R&D strategy in 1991. He said:

> Strongly held views based on belief rather than sound information still exert too much influence in health care. In some instances the relevant knowledge is available but not being used, in other situations additional knowledge needs to be generated from reliable sources.

Interestingly, Ellwood (1988) poses the theory that it could all be to do with timing. He quotes Sir Francis Darwin:

> In science the credit goes to the [one] who convinces the world, not to the [one] to whom the idea first occurs.

In other words, evidence about clinical effectiveness is largely missing because, until recently, clinicians have not been moved to address the problem. This theory is supported by the fact that evidence-based practice of clinical effectiveness is sparse in many medical and medically related fields (e.g. Altman and Bland, 1996; Ah-See et al., 1997). The amount of available research evidence is directly related to the amount of investment put into it.

Differences between efficacy, effectiveness and efficiency

It is important to distinguish between the terms 'treatment efficacy', 'treatment effectiveness' and 'treatment efficiency'. 'Treatment efficacy' involves the extent to which an intervention can be shown to be beneficial under experimental (optimal or ideal) conditions. Efficacy research 'documents that changes in performance are directly attributable to the treatment administered' (Campbell, 1995). Controlled clinical trials are investigations of treatment efficacy. 'Treatment effectiveness' involves the extent to which treatment can be shown to be beneficial under typical clinical conditions. Some treatment effectiveness studies attempt to validate treatment efficacy studies.

Treatment effectiveness studies may also attempt to address a variety of other questions – for example, the quality of the intervention, the patient's interaction with the therapist and the achievement of functional change (Campbell, 1995). However, in most speech and language therapy studies, the distinction between efficacy and effectiveness is not so distinct. Most good studies attempt to strike a balance between experimental control and clinical relevance. This dilemma is discussed in more detail in Chapter 2.

'Treatment efficiency' refers to the relative merits of one treatment compared with those of another. An efficient treatment means one in which maximum benefit is reached with minimum output (i.e. with respect to issues such as cost , the amount of time taken, etc.).

Clinical audit

Clinical audit is about reviewing and improving treatment in a systematic way. Research involves methodological investigation and aims to contribute to a body of knowledge. Audit is concerned with quality of care, examining whether actual practice matches standards set. Efficacy and effectiveness research focuses on identifying and proving what is best practice, whereas audit focuses on the actual implementation and evaluation of best practice. Implementing clinical audit generally involves a cyclical approach. This cycle comprises three stages: defining the expected level of quality; measuring and comparing actual practice against the expected levels; and taking action for improvement where any deficiencies are identified.

Evidence-based practice

Evidence-based practice is the judicious use of clinical evidence to help make an informed decision about the care for individual patients. It means 'integrating individual clinical expertise with the best available external clinical evidence from systematic research' (Sackett et al., 1995). Clinicians practising evidence-based skills will identify and apply the most efficacious interventions to maximise the quality of the probable result. Health-care commissioners have begun directly to introduce evidence on the effectiveness of intervention into the priority setting of health-care budgets (see Dixon et al., 1997). The principles of evidence-based practice provide a credible rationale for both the clinician and the health-care purchaser to structure an increasingly complex decision-making process. The search for the 'best' evidence possible involves the evaluation of the scientific evidence derived from research. Hierarchies of scientific evidence exist, based on the validity of different methodologies and the extent to which they reduce the likelihood of errors in the conclusions. An example is presented in Table 1.1.

Table 1.1 Classification of strength of evidence based on the quality of study methodology

Class I	Evidence provided by one or more well-designed, randomised controlled clinical trials
Class II	Evidence provided by one or more well-designed randomised clinical studies such as case–control, cohort studies and so forth
Class III	Evidence provided by expert opinion, randomised historical controls, or one or more case reports
Class IV	Evidence from well-designed, non-experimental studies from more than one centre or research group
Class V	Opinions provided by respected authorities, randomised historical controls, case reports, descriptive studies or reports from expert committees

From Moore et al. (1995)

The use of such classification systems may create significant problems for speech and language therapists, not just because our evidence base is so sparse, but also because existing evidence for most communication disorders (including voice disorders) falls largely into categories III–IV. As shown in Chapter 2, the voice literature has very few examples of clinical trials that would be classified in category I or II. However, there is some concern that the over-emphasis on the importance of randomised controlled trials (RCTs) hides the fact that other methods may be more suitable, depending on the question (Black, 1996). Also imposing the medical gold standard of the RCT may be inappropriate in many areas of rehabilitation and therapy research (Andrews, 1991; Gladman, 1991). Many important clinical questions cannot be realistically addressed by randomised controlled clinical trials. Some investigations may not be ethical, some investigations may be logistically impossible, some investigations may be too expensive, and some investigations may lack the ability to control all the necessary variables in order to draw meaningful conclusions. However, as a profession it is important that we use appropriate scientific methodology to produce the best evidence possible.

Systematic reviews

The use of systematic reviews is an essential part of the process of evidence-based practice; systematic reviews represent the most powerful means of collating evidence on the effectiveness of a particular treatment. It is a method used to 'identify, select and critically appraise relevant research' and to collect and analyse the data from individual studies (Mulrow and Oxman, 1997). Systematic reviews are one way of tackling the sheer volume of information that may exist for a particular treatment or intervention. They also provide a way of focusing on high-quality material, both published and unpublished, and drawing conclusions from previous work that may have proved inconclusive or conflicting (Mulrow, 1994). A systematic review requires (1) a formulation of a clear clinical question, (2) a search of the literature for relevant clinical papers and (3) an evaluation (critical appraisal) of the evidence for its validity and usefulness. Implementation of the findings into clinical decision-making is 'evidence-based practice'.

The need for involvement in establishing treatment effectiveness

The examination of clinical effectiveness requires a marriage of clinical and research activity. This is what makes the topic so exciting to some clinicians (and so frightening for others). Unfortunately, there is still the harmful opinion that clinical practice and rigorous research are mutually exclusive. It is an attitude that pits 'the researcher against the practitioner, and experimental control against informed clinical judgements' (Olswang, 1998). The opinion that research is not for clinicians is only reinforced when researchers do not address clinically relevant issues. But, by addressing clinical effectiveness, the researcher is also developing our scientific knowledge base; he or she is addressing phenomena with both theoretical and clinical applications. By asking clinical questions, by systematically documenting our clinical decision-making and by evaluating the outcomes of our treatment, we are simultaneously addressing theoretical issues.

Clinical practice needs clinical effectiveness research to inform it, to help in its improvement and development of its theoretical underpinnings and, ultimately, to ensure that it survives. Olswang (1993) states it all perfectly:

> For those of us driven by both clinical practice and theory, we have found our playground. Efficacy research allows us to function within our split interests – addressing practice and the needs of the individual while investigating theory and the underlying mechanisms of communication. What we need is further research with this two-pronged approach, advancing both our clinical and theoretical knowledge. Our profession and discipline indeed depends upon it. (page 131)

This book is meant to stimulate the speech and language therapist who works in the field of voice disorders to contribute to the debate about the effectiveness of our treatments. To many other speech and language therapy specialists, treatment effectiveness in voice disorders may seem obvious. Yet, critical evaluation of the literature and careful examination of the issues involved result in a far more complex picture.

The literature on voice therapy efficacy

The following chapters in this book discuss the main issues pertinent to measuring the effectiveness of voice therapy for voice-disordered patients. Each set of issues is debated in the context of the relevant literature. The studies were gathered from a variety of sources. Hillman et al. (1990), Carding and Horsley (1992), Verdolini-Marston et al. (1995), Enderby and Emmerson (1995) and Ramig and Verdolini (1998) were used as core articles. These papers identified 75% of the total studies found ($n = 24$). Cross-referencing from the original articles identified another seven papers. A computer-based literature search using Medline (*Index Medicus*) and Psych. Lit., using the key words 'voice therapy', 'speech therapy', 'dysphonia', 'aphonia', 'therapy efficacy', 'voice disorders' and 'voice clinic' identified a further six studies. All of the studies were concerned with voice or speech therapy for dysphonic patients with a large variety of voice disorders. Studies concerned with voice therapy for alaryngeal or oesophageal voice were not included. A total of 37 studies was found and these are listed in Table 1.2.

Table 1.2 Studies of voice therapy

Authors	Year	Type of study	Number of patients
Fisher and Logemann	1970	Single case	1
Strandberg et al.	1971	Single case	1
Shearer	1972	Single case	1
Zwitman and Calcaterra	1973	Single case	1
Brewer and McCall	1974	Single case	1
Holbrook et al.	1974	Single case	1
Rontal et al.	1975	Single case	1
Toohill	1975	Retrospective	77
Drudge and Phillips	1976	Prospective	3
Davis	1977	Single case	1
Prosek et al.	1978	Prospective	6
Stemple et al.	1980	Prospective	7
Bloch et al.	1981	Prospective	12
McIntyre	1981	Single case	1
Hayward and Simmons	1982	Prospective	64
Horsley	1982	Single case	1
Kay	1982	Retrospective	42
Ranford	1982	Single case	1
Bridger and Epstein	1983	Retrospective	109
Butcher and Elias	1983	Single case	1
Andrews et al.	1986	Prospective	10
D'Antonio et al.	1987	Single case	1
Beck	1988	Single case	1
Lancer et al.	1988	Retrospective	32
Kotby et al.	1991	Prospective	14
Koufman and Blalock	1991	Retrospective	157
Roy and Leeper	1991	Prospective	17
Ackerlund	1993	prospective	33
Kitzing and Ackerlund	1993	Prospective	28
Schneider	1993	Single case	1
Yamaguchi et al.	1993	Prospective	3
Blood	1994	Single cases	2
Fex et al.	1994	Prospective	10
Stemple et al.	1994	Prospective	35
Verdolini-Marston et al.	1995	Prospective	13
Bassiouny	1998	Prospective	+2
Carding et al.	1999	Prospective	45

Chapter 2
The importance of study design

Evaluation of the evidence of treatment efficacy involves the assessment of the extent to which an intervention can be shown to be beneficial under experimental (optimal or ideal) conditions. Efficacy research 'documents that changes in performance are directly attributable to the treatment administered' (Campbell, 1995). This is different from treatment effectiveness that is concerned with the extent to which treatment can be shown to be beneficial under typical clinical conditions. However, both types of study should aim to set up an experimental situation to measure the relationship between treatment and outcome. It is important to demonstrate that a change in patient performance is the direct result of treatment rather than from spontaneous improvement or from other interacting factors. There could be many reasons why a patient has improved and it may be misleading to assume that it was because of the treatment given. The cause and effect relationship can be examined by using a well-designed study methodology with the appropriate control of independent and dependent variables and accurate data interpretation.

Study methodology

Treatment efficacy/effectiveness research can employ many different types of methodological design. Studies of treatment outcome may ask many types of questions and therefore may require one of a number of methodological designs for the scientific structure of an investigation in order to answer them. Olswang (1998) observes that 'each design poses a different research question and these questions in turn shape the methodology'. Fineburg (1990) defined three basic methodologies in treatment efficacy research: experimental, quasi-experimental and non-experimental.

9

Experimental

These are studies that involve random or clearly stated assignment of patients to treatment and control groups. Randomized controlled clinical trials are considered to be the most powerful method of experimental research in this area (Frattali, 1998). This argument is disputed by clinical researchers who advocate the use of small-group or single-subject designs in order to examine more subtle effects of treatment.

Quasi-experimental

These are studies that involve non-random assignment of patients to treatment and non-treatment groups. These methodologies are often used because of the impracticality of true experimental design. Frattali (1998) suggests that there may be very good reasons why experimental design is not possible.

> Some experiments may not be ethical; some experiments are administra-
> tively and logistically impossible; some fail (i.e. due to loss of patients'
> numbers); and some experiments may lack the ability to control all
> variables in order to draw conclusions. (page 20)

A quasi-experimental methodology is one that falls short of meeting the requirements of the experimental research design but that employs a similar set of principles. The methodological dilemmas that underlie randomized clinical trials have resulted in a gradual acceptance of less rigorous designs. These include case-controlled retrospective studies and prospective cohort studies.

Non-experimental

These are studies that do not involve clear comparison groups. Non-experimental designs include case reports and expert opinion. In terms of proof of treatment efficacy these are, of course, the weakest methodological design. They are often subjective and are likely to lack experimental control.

Both single and multi-subject study designs can, however, have a significant role to play in investigating the effectiveness or efficacy of voice therapy. The choice of design is, to some extent, dependent on the question asked. If the question is 'Is my treatment effective for patient A?', then a single-case study may be appropriate. However, if the question is 'Are my treatment methods effective with patients with disorder A?', then the choice of a group study design may be more appropriate. There is one fundamental requirement that is pertinent to all treatment efficacy/effectiveness studies: it is necessary to demonstrate that treatment results in significantly more improvement than no treatment, and that the changes that occur are a function of therapy and not of other factors. In single-case studies, this problem can be addressed by using one of a number of designs, including: A–B–A; multiple baseline; and crossover design (see Kratochowill and Levin, 1994). In group studies the problems may be addressed by using no-treatment control conditions.

Single-case studies are often used to describe a voice therapy programme and to explore the treatment effect in depth. They are able to concentrate on individual observations that may be missed in a group study. Advocates of single-subject methodology argue that it is this uniqueness and diversity of the individual that necessitates the use of such designs. Furthermore, single-case study design is useful for generating hypotheses about the relationship between treatment and outcome. These hypotheses may then be tested in a group study design. Single-subject approaches also have the advantage that each subject serves as his or her own control, allowing the experimenter to escape the subject-matching problems and uncontrollable intersubject effects.

The main disadvantage of single-case studies relates to the difficulty of generalising the findings to a larger patient population. An apparently significant observation may or may not be idiosyncratic to the individual subject. There is a danger of interpreting individual variation as a significant effect. One way to deal with this is to produce a series of single-case studies to replicate individual findings. As most studies of efficacy in speech and language therapy have small sample sizes or use single-case design, replication (of the study method by the same or different clinicians on similar patients) is vital to provide verification and confirmation. Unfortunately, there are no examples of single-case studies in the voice therapy literature that have been replicated on a number of individuals.

Conversely, multi-subject designs have the obvious advantage of reporting treatment effects on larger numbers of patients. FitzGibbon (1986) takes the view that 'any effect which could be demonstrated in a case study could be more convincingly demonstrated in randomised controlled trials' (page 123). A significant effect in a group study may be seen to be more robust than the results from a single-case study. The larger the group study, the more convincing the effect may be. Randomized controlled trials are considered in medicine to be the most powerful evidence of the effects of treatment (Cochrane, 1972). This is because of their ability to randomize assignment of individuals to different treatment groups which is the best way of achieving a balance between groups for the known and unknown factors that influence outcome (Stephenson and Imrie, 1998). One aim of a group study is to be impartial, to ignore idiosyncratic behaviour, to discover underlying principles. Multi-subject studies also have the advantage of recording data for individual attention where appropriate, as well as for group results.

The main disadvantage of multi-subject or group design is concerned with the lack of homogeneity. Group studies need a certain degree of subject and treatment uniformity. Numerous variables may influence a patient's response to treatment. Multi-subject studies may be inappropriate when the potential variables are great. The impact of variables such as aetiological factors, intelligence, personality and psychosocial factors may influence treatment outcomes, but are difficult to control in a randomised study. Group studies attempt to control for these variables by employing inclusion and exclusion recruitment criteria or by randomizing them (and therefore balancing out their effect) across different treatment groups. Finally, group studies have been criticised for potentially missing important information about individual patients. However, as was mentioned above, this may not necessarily be the case if the data collection is sufficiently sensitive so that individual results can be discussed as well if appropriate.

Common flaws in study design

Despite the relative arguments for single-case versus group studies, it is important to note that a well-designed case series can be more meaningful than a poorly designed randomised controlled study. Rosenfeld (1995) describes a number of common flaws in study design. One should not only be careful to avoid these pitfalls when designing a study, but also be aware of them when critically evaluating other studies. The common design flaws are described briefly below. Many of these faults will be highlighted in the literature review of the voice therapy efficacy studies later in this chapter.

Hypothetical hypotheses

These are studies that leave the reader to guess the purpose of the study. Equally common is when the study hypothesis is formulated after collecting the data, and yet treated as if formulated before the start.

Schizophrenic study type

These are studies that think that they are something that they are not. For example; review articles that think that they are prospective studies or case reports that think that they are review articles. Rosenfeld (1995) states that most retrospective studies are commonly case series and most prospective studies appear as (but are not) randomised controlled studies.

Unrepresentative samples

These are studies that use a sample of patients that do not reflect the clinical population. It is not possible to generalise the results beyond the sample, unless the sample is truly representative of the intended population.

Clandestine controls

These involve creating a control group retrospectively or fortuitously (i.e. a group of patients happen not to have received the treatment that is being evaluated). Controls borrowed from other researchers or previous studies (historical controls) are also far from ideal (unless the recruitment and methodology of the two studies are identical).

Confounded outcomes

These are studies that analyse an outcome and then draw conclusions based on the result. It may be very misleading to assume that the outcome was the result of the intervention given. Confounding refers to an apparent association between two variables when none really exists. This is most commonly seen in the discussion of statistical correlations between variables. A correlation may or may not mean that the two variables are related in some way.

Independent variables

The independent variables of an efficacy or effectiveness study refer to those conditions that are manipulated to produce change – the differences among conditions that are likely to influence patient performance (and hence outcome). Manipulation of independent variables is at the heart of experimental design. It gives the clinician the opportunity to measure the effects of the variables without contamination of other major factors, which may influence treatment outcome. If a major variable (i.e. one that is likely to influence treatment outcome) is not manipulated, it should be controlled. In efficacy research, the major independent variables include subject/patient characteristics and the details of the treatment programme.

Control of subject characteristics is usually done by specifying inclusion and exclusion criteria for all patients in the study. This ensures that all patients share certain characteristics (i.e. non-smokers, no previous voice therapy, same laryngeal diagnosis). Of course, it may not be known which individual characteristics are the most important. Independent subject variables such as educational background, patient motivation, site of lesion, severity of disorder, etc., may be altered while the treatment programme remains the same in order to observe the change in outcome. If the outcome of treatment varies between patients with different characteristics, then the researcher has begun to make important discoveries about the treatment process and/or the nature of the disorder.

However, traditionally, treatment efficacy research involves manipulating the treatment variable. Treatments can be manipulated in a number of ways. Yeaton and Sechrest (1981) suggest that most efficacy studies manipulate either the *strength* and/or the *integrity* of treatment. Strength refers to the frequency and intensity of treatment. Integrity refers to the details of the treatment programme (i.e. the internal steps in the therapy programme, the amount of time spent at each step, the materials used, etc.).

It is not always possible or desirable to control every independent variable. The potential effect of less important variables can be minimised by either subject matching across treatment groups or by random allocation (which assumes that the effect of the variable is dissipated across the treatment groups). The more experimentally controlled a study is, the less it may reflect clinical practice. The researcher is therefore left with the dilemma of trying to design a study that will yield results that are experimentally sound and also clinically relevant.

Dependent variables

The dependent variables in an efficacy/effectiveness study are the outcome measures. The designer of the study needs to decide what to measure, how to measure and when to measure. The answers to these questions again lie in the nature of the original research question that is being proposed. If the question is very specific, such as 'Do breathing exercises improve air flow?', specific measures can be used (e.g. pneumotachography). If the question is more general, for example, 'Is treatment A better than treatment B?', then multiple measures should be employed to address the complexities of the disorder being treated (Olswang, 1998). However, regardless of the question, dependent variables must include measures that provide data, which can appropriately assess the nature and magnitude of the observed change.

An important consideration concerns the kind of data that should be collected from the dependent measures. One distinction that is commonly made is between quantitative and qualitative data. Quantitative data refer to numerical data: observable, countable, quantifiable. The advances in computer technology over the past 20 years have resulted in a large number of speech and voice instrumentation techniques (see Chapter 4), with the main advantage being that they produce quantitative data. Qualitative data are descriptive, observational and interpretative. Traditional voice measures, such as perceptual voice quality judgement and laryngoscopic examination, provide qualitative data. Here lies another significant dilemma for the clinician designing a voice treatment effectiveness/efficacy study. The techniques for the measurement of instrumental voice quality may provide more quantifiable data, which are seen to be less subjective, although the qualitative measurements may provide more useful information about how the voice sounds and functions. This dilemma is discussed further in Chapter 4.

Interpreting and analysing the data

The goal of efficacy/effectiveness research is to document significant change – change that is neither random nor unimportant (Bain and Dollaghan, 1991). Statistical analysis is concerned with changes in the dependent measures and whether or not these changes are likely to result from chance. Selecting appropriate statistical analyses is a vital but difficult task. Inappropriate selection can provide biased analyses of the data and thus yield invalid results. However, the most common cause for invalid results lies in basic flaws in the design of the study (i.e. bias in data collection, poor selection of outcome measurements, etc.).

A common problem with statistics in the voice therapy efficacy/effectiveness studies is how to deal with small patient numbers. Rosenfeld (1995) observes that authors either claim that their sample is 'too small for statistical analysis' or use inappropriate statistical tests. Rosenfeld suggests that the smaller the study sample, the more important statistical analysis is in order to make meaningful conclusions. He also states that, when sample sizes are modest (< 30 per group), non-parametric tests should be used unless the authors specifically prove the normal distribution of the data.

Another common problem is the assumption that statistical significance (a calculation of probability that the observed effect could result from chance) between an independent and dependent variable is proof of a relationship between them. The efficacy literature is full of spurious claims that a treatment is effective because a dependent variable has changed beyond accepted levels of chance. This, of course, may not be so, especially if we are not convinced of a valid link between the independent and dependent variable or if the design is so weak that the change may be caused by something completely different. Statistical analysis cannot assess causality and cannot measure clinical significance. These factors can be addressed only via the sense and logic of the study design.

Statistical analysis can provide powerful supporting evidence of treatment efficacy (and in most cases is absolutely necessary), but it can also disguise the truth (usually unintentionally). Intentional statistical confusion is amusingly called the 'dazzle phenomenon' by Darrell Huff, author of *How to Lie with Statistics* (1954):

> If you can't prove what you want to prove, demonstrate something else and pretend that they are the same thing. In the daze that follows the collision of statistics with the human mind, hardly anybody will notice the difference.

Previous voice therapy study designs

Single-case studies

There are a number of single-case studies published in the literature (Fisher and Logemann, 1970; Strandberg et al., 1971; Shearer, 1972; Zwitman and Calcaterra, 1973; Brewer and McCall, 1974; Holbrook et al., 1974; Rontal et al., 1975; Davis, 1977; MacIntyre, 1981; Horsley, 1982; Ranford, 1982; Butcher and Elias, 1983; D'Antonio et al., 1987; Beck, 1988; Schneider, 1993). In most cases, these are exploratory studies, which describe a new technique or test out a new hypothesis. They are not primarily intended to be studies of treatment efficacy. They are single-case studies (which provide an in-depth description of an individual) and are not single-subject designs (which experimentally investigate a treatment effect). None of the single-subject studies employed a methodological design (e.g. an A–B–A, crossover or multiple baseline design) in order to compare the effects of treatment with no treatment. Even though the single-case studies report successful outcomes for the particular therapy used, they should not be taken as evidence of treatment efficacy.

Blood (1994) reports on two patients with vocal nodules using experimental control conditions (a repeated A–B design). He describes the use of a computer-assisted voice therapy programme in the treatment of both patients. The experimental phases of the design are: (A) baseline; (B) voice therapy programme; (C) voice therapy programme and relaxation; and (D) follow-up. The actual ordering of the experimental phases was (A), (B), (B + C), (B), (B + C) and (D). Repeated baseline measures were made and post-therapy measures were repeated at 1, 2 and 3 months. Results indicate that both patients improved on a number of measurement parameters after therapy. This improvement was maintained at follow-up. This study illustrates the value of a carefully documented single-subject study design. As Howard (1986) points out, repeated single-subject designs can be valuable in furthering investigations into whether a treatment technique is equally effective with other patients with problems of a similar type. Replications of these studies (i.e. by different clinicians or on a number of similar single cases) would provide further evidence of treatment efficacy.

Retrospective studies

Bridger and Epstein (1983) reviewed the medical notes of 109 dysphonic patients who participated in a programme of voice therapy. They concluded that 56% of patients were ultimately considered 'cured' and a further 26% 'improved' after speech therapy involvement. In another retrospective study, Koufman and Blalock (1991) reported 71% success with 157 'voice abuse patients' and 63% success with 10 'habitually hoarse' cases. Lancer et al. (1988) collected patients' responses to a questionnaire and examined the treatment records in an attempt to evaluate the long-term outcome of a group of patients diagnosed as having hyperfunctional dysphonia. One group of patients had received surgical intervention only, whereas a second group had received surgical intervention and speech therapy. They concluded that patients who received a combination of both surgery and speech therapy benefited the most.

Toohill (1975) and Kay (1982) both present retrospective data on children with vocal nodules. Both studies report on relatively large numbers of patients ($n = 77$ and $n = 42$, respectively), and both divided the patients into subgroups to suggest a comparative study. Toohill (1975) identified four different treatment groups (including a no-treatment control group). The results indicated that the 'degree of cure' was equal across the three treatment groups and 'compared favourably' to the no-treatment control group. However, there was no randomised allocation of patients across groups. There was also no description of how the treatment groups differed. Kay (1982) also retrospectively subdivided his group of patients. He identified a number of patients with vocal nodules who had not received either surgical or speech therapy intervention. He used these patients as a control group. As there was no prospective random or controlled allocation of patients to the three patient groups, it is difficult to evaluate the importance of any identifiable differences between the groups. The studies by Toohill (1975) and Kay (1982) really represent clinical epidemiological studies that masquerade as quasi-experimental studies, because of the opportunity to break the data into subgroups and compare the results. As epidemiological studies they are very valuable, producing important data about incidence, onset characteristics and prognosis of the disorder.

Retrospective studies are descriptive examples of clinical experience but do not provide firm evidence of clinical efficacy. As they are retrospective reviews, the studies do not contain any control treatment conditions. The authors are therefore unable to determine whether the observed effects were the result of treatment or of a response from an uncontrolled variable. Retrospective studies, by their nature, are unable to plan a specific set of measurements at the pre- and post-treatment stages. As the data were collected retrospectively, the authors were unable to influence the nature or the consistency of how the outcomes (i.e. the patient reports) were documented in the notes.

Prospective group studies

In comparison to the retrospective reports, a number of authors have published prospective studies of dysphonia treatment efficacy. Here the authors have designed studies to ascertain the effects of their treatments and to control variables that might otherwise influence therapy outcomes. Wertz (1993) describes four main prospective group study 'types', which may be used in treatment efficacy studies. These are: single group design; comparison of treatments design; treatment versus no-treatment design; and comparison of treatments with a no-treatment control group.

Single-group design

Single-group design 'selects a group of patients, administers a pre-treatment outcome measure, provides treatment, repeats the pre-treatment outcome measure post-treatment and compares pre- and post-treatment performance. Improved performance post-treatment is interpreted as demonstrating the efficacy of treatment' (Wertz, 1993, page 63). A large majority of the published voice therapy efficacy group studies fall into this category. Drudge and Phillips (1976) and Hayward and Simmons (1982) provide examples of single group studies, but do not use a pre- and post-treatment set of measurements. Drudge and Phillips (1976) described the effect of a therapy programme used on three patients with vocal nodules. However, assessments were performed only at the pre-treatment stage, and therefore it was not possible to ascertain the level of change after treatment. Measurement of change relied on the qualitative comments of the otolaryngologist after indirect laryngoscopy, and the speech pathologist's comments concerning general 'improvement in voice quality'. Hayward and Simmons (1982) evaluated the use of group relaxation therapy in the treatment of 50 dysphonia patients. Conclusions about treatment efficacy were limited by the lack of pre- and post-treatment assessments. Evaluation concentrated on how valuable the patients thought the group sessions had been, and whether they were continuing to use their relaxation skills after the course had finished. Assessment of voice quality relied on descriptive comments by the patients. Evaluation of treatment efficacy was limited to general comments such as 'most [patients] were still having some voice loss' (Hayward and Simmons, 1982, page 2) or 'they were far less worried about it [their voice] and therefore less incapacitated' (page 3). Measuring the amount of change in voice quality after the group therapy programme was not undertaken.

Prosek et al. (1978) provided one of the earliest examples of a well-designed single-group study. Electromyographic (EMG) biofeedback voice therapy was evaluated in six patients who were judged to have excessive laryngeal tension phonation. The frequency distribution of EMG activity was collected for all six patients pre- and post-treatment. The results suggested that the treatment reduced EMG activity in three patients with a concomitant improvement in voice quality. The three other patients did not appear to improve with the therapy technique. Bloch et al. (1981) describe the results of a single group of 12 patients with vocal fold contact granuloma. All of the patients received a well-described programme of voice therapy. The results of the treatment were evaluated by a laryngologist, a speech therapist and the patient him- or herself. The success rate of voice therapy was stated at 71% (12 of 17 cases) or 100% (eliminating 5 of 17 cases who terminated voice therapy very early).

There have been several more recent single-group design studies that have also provided valuable evidence of voice therapy efficacy (Kotby et al., 1991; Roy and Leeper, 1991; Yamaguchi et al., 1993; Fex et al., 1994). Yamaguchi et al. (1993) used several acoustic parameters to evaluate a 'pushing exercise programme' to correct for glottal incompetence. However, the authors reported on only three patients in this study and hoped to publish a larger series soon after. Kotby et al. (1991) examined the efficacy of the accent method of voice therapy (Bergendal-Fex, 1976) in 28 patients with a variety of vocal pathologies (including functional, minor pathological, paralytic and neurogenic aetiology). An improvement in the patient's voice condition was reported in 25 of the 28 subjects. Patients with some laryngeal pathologies (i.e. hyperfunctional dysphonia, $n = 7$) provided more conclusive evidence of improvement over a variety of perceptual and instrumental measurements in comparison to other pathologies (i.e. vocal nodules). Roy and Leeper (1991) measured the effects of a manual reduction technique for laryngeal musculoskeletal tension, as a treatment of functional voice disorder. The voice quality of all 17 patients in this study improved after voice therapy. The authors recognised that their study reported on only short-term voice improvement and that objective long-term maintenance data were needed. However, by virtue of the fact that almost no empirical evidence exists in the research literature to support any alternative therapy approaches, the authors concluded that these reduction techniques 'deserve[d] serious consideration by practising voice clinicians' (Roy and Leeper, 1991, page 248). Fex et al. (1994) studied 10 'functional' dysphonia patients treated with voice therapy using the 'accent method' (Bergendal-Fex, 1976). A range of assessments was used at both the pre- and post-treatment stages. Fex et al. concluded that their treatment method was effective in all 10 patients.

These single-group studies all employed a design in which each patient was his or her own control and in which a pre-treatment baseline set of measurements was taken before therapy started. In some cases, there was also evidence of prospective control of patient and treatment independent variables. For example, Bloch et al. (1981) used a specific diagnostic inclusion criterion (contact granuloma) and limited the study sample to males from upper-middle socioeconomic classes. The voice treatment programme was also described in detail and was administered with consistency across the study subjects. However, single-group studies do not use no-treatment control groups. It is therefore difficult to indicate whether the improvements noted in these studies are a result of the treatment or of another uncontrolled factor(s). Single-group studies cannot answer this question.

Comparison of treatment design

Comparison of treatment design 'assigns patients randomly to one treatment or another, collects pre-treatment performance on an outcome measure, administers the specified treatments, repeats the pre-treatment outcome measures post-treatment, and compares improvement between the treatment groups to determine whether one treatment resulted in more improvement than the other' (Wertz, 1993, page 63). The comparison of treatment design is limited to demonstrating whether a treatment is the same as, better than or worse than the other. It will not demonstrate whether either is efficacious. It is interesting to note that very few studies have prospectively compared the effects of more than one treatment approach. This is surprising, given that there is a range of different therapy approaches available for the treatment of voice disorders.

As mentioned earlier, Toohill (1975) presented data on 77 children with vocal nodules who received four differential therapy programmes (no-treatment, $n=19$; school-based speech therapy, $n=33$; private speech therapy, $n=13$; and social work family counselling, $n=12$). Also Kay (1982) presented data on 42 children with vocal nodules who had received no treatment ($n=13$), surgical intervention ($n=13$) or speech therapy ($n=16$). Although the results from these two studies attempted to differentiate between the relative benefits of the different treatment modalities, they do not represent prospective comparison of treatment studies. The patients were not prospectively or randomly assigned to the treatment/no-treatment groups. It is likely that there were a number of important reasons why a patient was placed in a particular group (i.e. too ill for surgery, failed to attend speech therapy) and these factors may have a significant impact on the treatment outcomes.

Andrews et al. (1986) compared EMG biofeedback and relaxation techniques using five matched pairs of patients diagnosed as having 'hyperfunctional dysphonia'. The results showed that the voices of all patients in both treatment groups showed significant difference from their pre-treatment state. Both EMG biofeedback therapy and relaxation therapy were reported to have improved the voice quality of the patients in the study. Without a no-treatment condition, this type of study is able to compare only the relative value of the two different treatment programmes. It is not able to examine whether either treatment is any more effective than no treatment.

Bassiouny (1998) reported on 42 patients with a variety of vocal pathologies who were distributed randomly into two groups. Patients in group I were given the full aspect of the accent method of voice therapy, i.e. voice hygiene plus the accent exercises to correct faulty vocal technique. Patients in group 2 received only voice hygiene advice. Voice evaluations were made at pre-test (baseline), mid-test and the termination of intervention/therapy (post-test). Assessments included a subjective rating of voice quality (clinician and patient) and a number of instrumental measures (laryngo-video-stroboscopy, aerodynamic measures, acoustic analysis and inverse filtering measures). The difference in improvement between the two groups was statistically significant for most assessments in favour of group I, who received the full accent method programme. In addition, there were significant improvements in patients in group 1 in certain items specific for the various aetiological categories.

Treatment versus no-treatment group design

The treatment versus no-treatment group design constitutes 'the classical clinical trial designed to determine treatment's efficacy' (Wertz, 1993, page 64). This type of clinical trial requires random assignment of patients who meet selection criteria into treatment and no-treatment groups. Typically

> . . . pre-treatment performance on an outcome measure is collected; the treatment groups are treated with the specified treatment and the no-treatment group is followed up. At the end of the treatment trial, the outcome measure is re-administered and improvement is compared between groups. (Wertz, 1993, page 65)

In their review of the literature in 1995, Wilson et al. could find examples of a randomised controlled group study to evaluate the effectiveness of voice therapy.

Stemple et al. (1980) compare EMG readings of laryngeal muscle tension in 21 normal subjects and 7 with vocal nodules. There was a statistically significant difference in muscle tension EMG between the normal and pathological subjects. However, the normal subjects do not, of course, constitute a no-treatment control group. The subjects with vocal fold nodules significantly reduced their EMG levels after treatment (EMG biofeedback training), but these results cannot be compared with a no-treatment or different treatment group. The treatment of the seven pathological patients represents a single-group design. Stemple et al. (1994) evaluated the efficacy of 'vocal function exercises' as a method of improving voice production. The 35 adult women were randomly divided into experimental, placebo and control groups. This design represents a double-blind, placebo-controlled design. However, the subjects all had normal voices. The authors used subjects with normal voices in order to establish measurable benefits from the voice therapy programme. Their intention was then to apply the same techniques to a pathological population should the exercises prove beneficial. For this reason, the study does not directly address the effectiveness of voice therapy on dysphonic patients, although the study constitutes an important preliminary study on which clinical studies may be based.

Verdolini-Marston et al. (1995) also published a preliminary study of the effectiveness of treatment for laryngeal nodules. Thirteen women with vocal nodules were assigned to either one of two treatment groups or a no-treatment control group. Assignment to the groups was not random, but made on the basis of severity ratings in an attempt to control this variable. The authors considered severity of presentation (at videostroboscopic examination) to be a potentially important factor in determining treatment outcome. A number of measures were taken before treatment, one day after the termination of treatment and then 2 weeks post-treatment. Statistically significant differences were shown between the results of the treatment groups and those of the control group. Thus, benefit from therapy was shown. However, there was no difference between the results of the two different treatment programmes ('confidential' voice therapy and 'resonance' voice therapy). The clarity of the design methodology of this study produces sound evidence of treatment efficacy even though the subject numbers were small.

Carding et al. (1999) describe a prospective control group study of 45 patients with non-organic dysphonia. The patients were assigned in rotation to one of three treatment groups. Patients in group 1 received no treatment and acted as a control group. Patients in groups 2 and 3 received a programme of 'indirect' therapy and 'direct + indirect' therapy, respectively. A range of qualitative and quantitative measures was carried out on all patients before and after treatment to evaluate change in voice quality over time. Results revealed a statistically significant difference between the three treatment groups for voice severity ratings, electrolaryngograph and shimmer measurements, and on ratings provided by a patient questionnaire. However, other measures (*Fo* analysis, jitter and signal-to-noise ratio measurements) failed to show significant differences between the three groups. Most of the patients (86%) in the control group showed no significant change in any of the measures. Some patients (46%) in group 2 showed significant changes in voice quality. Of 15 patients in group 3, 14 (93%) showed significant changes in voice quality. Enderby and Emmerson (1995, page 162) state that the strength of the design of this study 'offers good evidence that voice therapy is successful in treating this group of patients'.

Statistical evidence

As stated earlier, a study of treatment effectiveness must demonstrate that the changes that occur are not the probable result of 'chance'. Sound evidence of efficacy must therefore employ appropriate statistical measures (which simply state the level at which the results are above the likelihood of chance). A study with a good methodological design is of limited value if the results are not subjected to valid statistical analysis.

Only 48% of the studies that have been mentioned in the previous sections of this chapter employed any statistical analysis to support their evidence of clinical effectiveness. One main reason for this is the common use of qualitative data, which are often descriptive and not numerical. Several studies have attempted to quantify the qualitative data by counting patients who fall into a specified descriptive category, i.e. 'completely free of symptoms' (Bloch et al., 1981) or 'considered cured' (Toohill, 1975). This quantification is usually expressed by percentages (e.g. 80% of patients were judged to have improved, etc.). The last 10 years had seen a large increase in the use of instrumental voice measurement techniques (Ramig and Verdolini, 1998). This has inevitably resulted in more quantifiable data, which have lent themselves to mathematical analysis. A large majority of studies in the 1990s use more appropriate statistical analyses.

Conclusion: solving some study design problems

Hillman et al. (1990) reviewed the treatment efficacy studies for non-organic voice disorders up to their year of publication. They noted the following problems with most of the study designs in the literature:

1. No control group within which spontaneous improvement may be observed and against which a treatment group could be compared.
2. Absence of a pre-treatment baseline against which the post-treatment measurements could be judged.
3. No experimental control of factors that may influence the effect of treatment.
4. A lack of internal consistency in the methodology of the study (i.e. where all the patients in the study did not receive the same set of measurements at all stages of assessment).
5. Limited results as a consequence of insufficient numbers of patients – some studies had good designs but were only used on one or two patients.

The review in this chapter reaches similar conclusions even though it involved an evaluation of voice therapy treatment for both non-organic and organic voice disorders, and included published studies up to and including 1998. There is no doubt that there has been an improvement in the quality of the voice therapy efficacy research over the past 10 years. We now have a number of group studies that provide some evidence of a positive treatment effect (Kotby et al., 1991; Roy and Leeper, 1991; Yamaguchi et al., 1993; Fex et al, 1994; Verdolini-Marston et al., 1995; Carding et al., 1999). These studies are largely successful in providing pre- and post-treatment baseline data to measure and document change accurately. They also often attempt to control variables that might otherwise affect treatment outcomes. It is not possible, of course, to control for all of the potential variables that might affect treatment outcomes, the major variables in this type of study usually being patient specific (Wertz, 1993). The most common and most practical way of controlling some of these variables is to use patient-selection criteria. Contaminating influences that are not controlled in this way may be minimised by randomly allocating patients across different treatment groups.

Only Verdolini-Marston et al. (1995) and Carding et al. (1999), however, attempt to use a no-treatment control condition within which spontaneous improvement could be observed, and against which treatment conditions could be compared. There is, of course, an ethical issue in using a no-treatment condition in a study design of treatment effectiveness. Prevention of access to treatment for a significant period of time can only really be considered ethical when there is genuine uncertainty about which treatment to offer. Conversely, failure to examine genuine uncertainty about treatment value through well-designed studies could also be considered unethical, because it allows ineffective treatments to continue unabated. A no-treatment phase (either within an individual or a group study) may be considered the same as being on a waiting list for treatment.

In summary, the design limitations identified by Hillman et al. in 1990 still apply to most studies of voice therapy effectiveness. However, it is possible to design a study that can overcome many of these fundamental methodological problems. A suggested approach to the design of an efficacy study for voice-disordered patients is shown in Figure 2.1.

1. Define the group of patients to be examined (e.g. by diagnosis, by occupation)

2. Establish a set of selection criteria in order to control for variables that may influence treatment outcome (e.g. onset time of dysphonia, patient's motivation). Exclude all patients who do not fulfil these criteria

3. Establish a no-treatment condition against which treatment effects can be compared. Randomly assign all patients to treatment and no-treatment groups

4. Assess all patients who enter the study to establish a baseline for each patient before treatment commences. A variety of assessments that measure different aspects of the voice disorder would be recommended

5. Define the treatment approaches so as to facilitate replication. Define the criteria by which the outcomes of the treatment will be judged (e.g. that the voice will be judged to be within normal limits by a group of expert listeners)

6. After treatment, reassess all patients in the study using the same techniques as before. This reassessment should take place immediately after the course of treatment is completed and at a review appointment (e.g. one month later)

7. Compare patient's pre- and post-assessments to establish the degree of improvement. Compare the results of the patients who received treatment with the patients in the no-treatment control group

Figure 2.1 A study design to measure treatment efficacy in voice-disordered patients.

Chapter 3
Defining some major independent variables

Olswang (1998) observed that the major independent variables in an efficacy study are patient characteristics (i.e. diagnosis, age, voice quality) and treatment programme details (i.e. frequency and content of voice therapy programme). As it is these variables that are experimentally manipulated in a treatment study, they require careful definition. However, in some cases, there is no definition of these terms. Where there are definitions, they are (1) not widely accepted, (2) in conflict with each other or (3) too vague to be of value. In an area where we are 'mired in a terminological swamp' (Perkins, 1985), there is a need to explain and define almost all the terminology that we use. Unfortunately, previous studies of voice therapy efficacy often have not defined important aspects of their study. This has led to a confusion about how relevant a particular study is and how it can be compared with other studies.

Defining subject/patient characteristics

Previous voice therapy efficacy studies have defined their subject group according to (1) aetiological factors, (2) perceptual (voice quality) factors or (3) diagnostic category.

A number of studies have chosen to select patients for their study on the basis of the *cause* of their dysphonia. Holbrook et al. (1974) describe a number of single cases, all of whom have a dysphonia caused by vocal abuse. Prosek et al. (1978) and Stemple et al. (1980) both describe group studies of patients in whom laryngeal hyperfunction is described as the cause of their voice problems. Andrews et al. (1986) matched pairs of patients with similar aetiological factors (i.e. predominantly psychogenic, from either occupational demands on the voice or exposure to environmental irritants). Yamaguchi et al. (1993) reported

27

on 29 patients with glottal incompetence caused by either paralysis or sulcus vocalis (a 'furrow' along the body of the vocal fold ligament – Hirano, 1981). This uniformity with respect to the *cause* of the dysphonia meant that the authors could evaluate a particular voice therapy technique to remedy the condition.

Other studies have chosen to select patients according to a specific abnormality of perceptual voice quality. Wolfe and Steinfatt (1987) examined a group of dysphonic patients who were classified into 'predominantly breathy' and 'predominantly hoarse' voice types. Imaizumi (1986) studied 98 patients who had been judged as having 'rough' voices, as opposed to 'breathy' or 'strained' ones (using Hirano's GRBAS scale – Hirano, 1981). The main advantage of this was that the authors were able to select a measurement technique to match the voice quality type. For example, use of jitter measurements to monitor the progress of 'predominantly breathy' voices and shimmer to monitor 'predominantly harsh' voices may provide relevant objective data.

However, most of the previous studies have selected their patients on the basis of laryngeal diagnosis. This creates a problem because there is no standard classification system for diagnosis of dysphonia. Traditionally, 'organic' laryngeal pathology is considered to be more accurately diagnosed and precisely defined than 'non-organic' voice disorders (Dikkers and Schutte, 1991). It is not surprising therefore that the most common diagnostic category investigated is vocal fold nodules (Fisher and Logemann, 1970; Shearer, 1972; Brewer and McCall, 1974; Toohill, 1975; Kay, 1982; Verdolini-Marston et al., 1995). The number of studies of patients with vocal fold nodules does not reflect the relative prevalence of the condition, but instead reflects the ease and agreement with which it is diagnosed. There is, however, evidence that even the diagnosis of benign organic laryngeal pathology suffers from poor definition and inaccurate classification (Dikkers and Schutte, 1991).

The definition of the diagnostic category is most problematic in the area of 'non-organic' voice disorders. For example, the voice therapy efficacy studies listed in Table 3.1 are all concerned with the treatment of dysphonic patients in whom there is no organic pathology to explain the disorder, but they do not all use the same diagnostic terms.

A closer review of the literature of non-organic dysphonia illustrates the difficulties that may occur when authors use different diagnostic categories and labels to define their subject group. In some of these studies, the chosen term has not been defined at all; in others it has been defined incompletely. In some reports, the authors describe the term in detail, but these definitions may vary between different studies.

Andrews et al. (1986) described the treatment of 10 'hyperfunctional dysphonia' patients, but did not define the term any further. It is,

Table 3.1 Terms that are used in the literature to mean 'dysphonia in the absence of organic pathology'

Terminology	Authors
Functional dysphonia	Rontal et al. (1975)
	Airainer and Klingholz (1993)
	Fex et al. (1994)
Psychogenic dysphonia	Strandberg et al. (1971)
	Horsley (1982)
	Hayward and Simmons (1982)
Mechanical dysphonia	McIntyre (1981)
Functional voice disorder	Koufman and Blalock (1982)
	Bridger and Epstein (1983)
	Roy and Leeper (1991)
Hyperfunctional voice	Drudge and Phillips (1976)
Hyperfunctional dysphonia	Andrews et al. (1986)
	Hillman et al. (1989)
Non-organic dysphonia	Ackerlund (1993)

therefore, unclear what types of dysphonia may or may not be included within this diagnostic category. This is in contrast to the work of Hillman et al. (1989) who also used the term 'hyperfunctional dysphonia'. In this case, the authors presented a theoretical background to justify the use of the term and clearly differentiated it from 'hypofunctional dysphonia'.

There are other examples in the literature of different studies using the same term, but this definition is not synonymous across them. Bridger and Epstein (1983), for example, defined 'functional dysphonia' as an impairment of voice 'in the absence of visible mucosal disease, and in spite of full vocal cord movement and complete closure on phona-tion' (page 1145). This is different to the definition proposed by Koufman and Blalock (1982) where a voice disorder is called 'functional':

> . . . when it is primarily due to abuse and misuse of the anatomically and physiologically intact vocal apparatus. The underlying cause may be obscure or obvious, but prolonged abuse may result in the development of nodules, polyps, ulcers or granulomas of the vocal cords. (page 372)

Therefore it is clear that these two studies were examining different groups of patients.

Conversely, there are examples in the literature where different terms have been used, but are being used as synonyms by different authors. For example, McIntyre (1981) and Drudge and Phillips (1976) used the diagnostic labels 'mechanical dysphonia' and 'hyperfunctional voice' respectively. However, both described these to mean dysphonia caused by excessive laryngeal tension and effort during phonation, with resultant prolonged voice misuse. Therefore, these studies examined the same patient population despite using a different diagnostic label.

Ackerlund (1993) described a study of treatment efficacy for patients with 'non-organic dysphonia'. He described it as 'an insufficiency of the voice where microlaryngoscopy does not reveal any pathology' (page 102). The major difficulty with this term (and with Ackerlund's definition) is the definition of the actual division between non-organic and organic voice pathology (Fawcus, 1986). For example, the development of nodules, polyps and granulomas of the vocal folds are often seen as the final product of prolonged inappropriate use of the laryngeal musculature during phonation (Koufman and Blalock, 1982). A voice disorder that started as a non-organic problem may result in the development of an organic lesion on the vocal folds. This division between organic and non-organic dysphonia is important because decisions about treatment may rest on how a vocal condition is labelled (Dikkers and Schutte, 1991).

It is apparent from this that no one diagnostic term is clearer than any other. With this degree of disagreement in the literature, it is important to define carefully the diagnostic term that is selected. This definition will almost certainly vary from some other previously published definitions.

Defining the therapy programme

There are many different therapy techniques for treatment of patients with dysphonia. The therapy programmes that are described in the literature generally fall into two main categories: therapy that concentrates on the psychosocial aspects and therapy that concentrates on the mechanical/physical aspects (Carding et al., 1999). However, these categories are not mutually exclusive; therapy that concentrates on a particular aspect of a voice problem may also allude to or influence other aspects. Within either of these general approaches to treatment, there are a number of accepted therapy techniques that are available to the clinician. A list of commonly used voice therapy techniques is shown in Table 3.2.

There has been very little research into why a clinician chooses a particular method of therapy for an individual patient. The choice is likely to be explained by a combination of the theoretical orientation of the clinician (i.e. whether they consider the problem to be predominantly

Table 3.2 A list of commonly used voice therapy techniques for treating dysphonia patients

Indirect treatment techniques

1. Vocal rest programme (Prater and Swift, 1984)
2. Patient education (Aronson, 1985)
    Explanation of the problem (Olsen, 1972)
3. Reassurance (Greene and Mathieson, 1989)
4. General relaxation (Martin, 1987)
5. Counselling (Aronson, 1985; Brumfit, 1986)
    Non-directive counselling (Rogers, 1981)
6. Auditory training (Boone, 1983; Fawcus, 1986)
7. Elimination of abuse/misuse (Boone, 1982; Johnson, 1985)
8. Voice diary (Prater and Swift, 1984)
9. Vocal hygiene programme (Wilson, 1987)
10. A 10-step outline for voice abuse (Wilson, 1987)
11. Avoidance of laryngeal irritants (Greene and Mathieson, 1989)
12. Environmental awareness (Prater and Swift, 1984)
13. Voice conservation advice (Greene and Mathieson, 1989)
14. Hierarchy analysis (Boone, 1983; adapted from Wolpe, 1973)

Direct treatment techniques

1. Specific laryngeal relaxation (Jacobsen, 1934; Martin, 1987)
2. Yawn–sigh method (Boone, 1982)
3. Chewing technique (Froeschels, 1952)
4. Altering tongue position (Boone, 1982)
5. Diaphragmatic breathing (Greene, 1980; Martin, 1987)
6. Coordination of breathing with phonation (Martin 1987)
7. Establishing and maintaining appropriate laryngeal tone (Boone, 1982)
8. Pitch variation and control (Boone, 1982)
9. Reduction of vocal loudness (Prater and Swift, 1984)
10. Elimination of hard glottal attack (Moncur and Bracket, 1974; Martin, 1987)
11. Establishing optimal pitch (Cooper, 1973; Boone 1983)
12. Voice 'placing' (Perkins, 1981; Boone, 1983)
13. Developing optimal resonance (Zailouk, 1963; Fawcus, 1986)
14. Maintenance and generalisation of optimal phonatory control (Boone, 1983)
15. Laryngeal manipulation (Roy and Leeper, 1991)
16. Accent method (Bergendal-Fex, 1976)
17. Pushing exercises for glottal incompetence (Yamaguchi et al., 1993)
18. Confidential voice therapy (Verdolini-Marston et al., 1995)
19. Resonant voice therapy (Verdolini-Marston et al., 1995)

psychological or mechanical), the clinician's perception of what is most appropriate to the patient, and what the patient is most likely to respond to. This means that voice therapy may take different forms in different studies. Indeed, the voice therapy for different patients in the same study may be dissimilar (Carding and Horsley, 1992).

With this degree of variability, it is important that the treatment programme is described in detail. In some of the efficacy studies, the therapy intervention has been carefully described, whereas in others, it has not been described at all. In the case of the latter studies, the emphasis would be more on assessing the value of a particular voice measurement rather than on describing a therapy programme. In the case of the studies that describe treatment, it should be done in detail so that it can be fully understood and replicated.

Most of the single-case studies of voice therapy provide detailed descriptions of a particular therapy programme. For example, McIntyre (1981) described each individual step of an outpatient treatment programme for a 'straight forward case of mechanical dysphonia'. This included details of exercises in supine relaxation, deep central breathing, expiratory breath control for phonation, gentle attack voicing and reinforcement of new voicing patterns. Horsley (1982) described a programme of hypnosis and self-hypnosis in the treatment of a patient with psychogenic dysphonia. The description included the method of induction and the detailed instructions that were given to the patient in order to facilitate a state of deep relaxation. Strandberg et al. (1971) describe the treatment procedure used with a 40-year-old woman with psychogenic hoarseness. The detailed therapy programme included training in deep muscle relaxation, instruction in phonation in controlled vowel contexts and gradual re-introduction of normal voice quality. These single-case studies provide valuable information about the implementation of a therapy programme by an individual clinician.

Several of the prospective group studies also described their therapy programme in detail. Drudge and Phillips (1976) detailed the therapy procedures used on three patients with vocal nodules. One main purpose of their study was to describe the learning process involved in shaping the changed behaviour of the three dysphonic patients. A 31-step programme for remediation of 'voice-abuse dysphonia' was listed. The programme was designed to shape behaviour through a series of increasingly difficult steps. Each step of the programme was intended to lead towards the achievement of one of four major goals: elimination of vocal abuse, easy initiation of phonation, increase in clear phonation, and increase in loudness without increase in laryngeal tension.

Verdolini-Marston et al. (1995) also describe their treatment programmes for patients with vocal nodules. They evaluated the use of two different therapy approaches: 'confidential voice therapy' and 'resonant voice therapy'. All patients received instruction in general vocal hygiene before being assigned to their treatment group. 'Confidential voice therapy' focuses on the elicitation of a minimal intensity, low effort and slightly breathy mode of phonation in speaking confidentially at close range. 'Confidential voice therapy' is considered to be particularly useful during the initial stages of treatment for maximum early reduction of vocal fold lesions as a result of habitual hyperfunctional voice use. 'Resonant therapy' involves vibratory sensations on the alveolar ridge and other facial areas during phonation. These sensations are thought to arise from a relative acoustic tuning of the supraglottal cavities with the glottal source spectrum (Verdolini-Marston et al., 1995).

Prosek et al. (1978) and Stemple et al. (1980) both describe the use of electromyographic (EMG) biofeedback in the treatment of patients with hyperfunctional voice disorders. The first study used a noise generator to alert the patient to excessive muscle tension. This enabled the patient to have simultaneous biofeedback during phonation tasks. The second study used a more latent biofeedback device, which calculated a general muscle-tension score of the laryngeal area after the speaking of phonetically balanced vocal tasks. Both techniques demonstrated that patients could voluntarily reduce the degree of laryngeal muscle tension when aided by the EMG biofeedback devices.

Yamaguchi et al. (1993) evaluated a 'pushing exercise programme' to correct for functional glottal incompetence. The pushing method is a voice therapy technique designed to reduce glottal inefficiency by increasing glottal closure. This method uses the principle that, in order to build up thoracic pressure, it is necessary to close the larynx. Thus, the technique takes advantage of the synchronous responsive adduction of the vocal folds when the neck and the upper arms are consciously strained in any manner that requires intrathoracic pressure build-up. The preliminary results demonstrated improvements in the three patients reported on.

Roy and Leeper (1991) measured the effects of a manual reduction technique for laryngeal musculoskeletal tension as a treatment of functional voice disorder. This treatment approach involved 'kneading the laryngeal musculature and lowering the position of the larynx in the neck ' (page 243). The technique includes encircling the hyoid bone with the thumb and middle finger, and exerting light pressure in a circular motion. A similar procedure is repeated in the thyrohyoid space and over the superior borders of the thyroid cartilage. Seventeen 'functional dysphonia' patients were treated using this approach.

Fex et al. (1994) studied 10 functional dysphonia patients treated with voice therapy using the 'accent method' (Bergendal-Fex, 1976).

This method focuses on developing a relaxed body position, abdominal breathing and a natural optimal pitch. Sustained phonation with variations in loudness (accents) is used, demonstrated first by the therapist and then copied by the patient.

In other studies, the authors have described in detail the assessment and measurement of dysphonic patients, but have not included the description of the voice therapy treatment programme. Davis (1977) analysed a range of acoustic features in a patient receiving voice therapy after surgical removal of undifferentiated vocal fold oedema. Davis used acoustic measurements to monitor progress throughout the treatment programme, and to demonstrate the successful outcome of therapy. However, details of the treatment programme were not given. Schneider (1993) described a range of perceptual and instrumental techniques to track voice change in a 27-year-old woman with 'hyperfunctional dysphonia'. The intensive vocal hygiene therapy programme was not described at all. Hayward and Simmons (1982) evaluated the use of group relaxation therapy in the treatment of 33 dysphonia patients. Each group's therapeutic direction varied according to the needs of the individuals within that group. They did not document the treatment programme of each member of each group individually.

The literature demonstrates that there are many different voice therapy techniques for the treatment of dysphonia patients. The voice therapist selects a treatment programme that reflects their perception of the cause of the problem and that is appropriate to the needs and expectations of the individual. This point is illustrated in the description of voice therapy for 17 patients with vocal fold granuloma (Bloch et al., 1981). The authors stated that their voice therapy methods 'varied according to each patient's needs' (page 49). They described a general regimen of voice treatment, but were keen to point out that some aspects were more pertinent to some patients than to others. 'When there was evidence of excessive hard glottal attack, the patient was made aware of this in an effort to eliminate them' (page 49). Most clinicians combine a variety of therapy techniques in order to find the most suitable approach for any individual patient (Boone and McFarlane, 1988). This means that, in a group study, the therapy programme may not be identical for each patient. In such a situation it is important to document the intervention for each patient.

Defining what 'effectiveness' means

'Effectiveness' is a difficult term to define. The interpretation of its meaning influences the design of the study, the definition of the independent and dependent variables, and the choice of outcome measures. There is a discussion of the difference between 'efficacy' and 'effectiveness' in Chapter 1. However, a definition of 'effectiveness' should incorporate a number of issues: first, treatment effectiveness should be linked to the goals of the intervention; second, measurement of effectiveness should be multi-dimensional and as comprehensive as possible; finally, studies about treatment effectiveness should be concerned with the investigation of the benefits of intervention in a clinically relevant setting. These points are all discussed further below.

Goal-specific effectiveness

Treatment can be said to be effective if it reaches the goals that it set out to attain. An important stage in defining 'effective' treatment is therefore to define the specific goal(s) of the therapy against which the actual outcome can be judged. The clearer the therapy goals, the easier it is to determine whether or not these goals have been achieved. The clearer the goals, the easier it is to decide on the outcome measures. A study that does not state the goals of treatment cannot be clear about what the outcome measures are. This, of course, allows the authors to select the outcome measures that show a significant change after therapy and discard those that do not. This is termed a 'false-positive' response.

Some studies state clearly the criteria on which the success of treatment will be judged. For example, Bloch et al. (1981) stated that successful voice therapy for patients with contact granuloma was when the laryngologist judged that there was complete disappearance of the vocal fold lesion, when the speech and language therapist judged that full voice recovery and normal manner of phonation had occurred, and when the patient judged him- or herself to be completely free of symptoms. Studies that examine treatment of patients with discrete laryngeal pathology caused by voice abuse/misuse or habitual vocal hyperfunction have an in-built success criterion. Effective treatment should result in elimination of or at least significant reduction in the size of the lesion. This may explain the disproportionate number of studies that have examined the efficacy of treatment for vocal nodules. With less definite laryngeal diagnosis (i.e. 'glottal incompetence' – Yamaguchi et al., 1993 – or 'non-organic dysphonia' – Carding et al., 1999), the situation is much less clear. In these studies, it may not be possible to document any physical changes in the larynx and so effectiveness must be judged against specific treatment aims.

Comprehensive effectiveness

Effectiveness can mean different things to different people. A study that considers effectiveness from one perspective only may be considered limited or even potentially biased. There are several examples of efficacy studies in which a single instrumental measurement technique has been used to document the effects of voice therapy. These studies have published the evidence of treatment efficacy based on the statistical difference between instrumental measurement values. If the measurements showed a statistically significant change, the authors concluded that the treatment was effective. In these cases, statistical significance has been confused with treatment effectiveness.

Cooper (1974) provided an early example of using Yanagihara's (1967a) spectrographic classification system to evaluate 27 dysphonia patients with a variety of laryngeal diagnoses. All of the patients' voices demonstrated characteristics of abnormal voice quality described as 'hoarse', which could be classified as spectrographically abnormal before therapy began. After therapy, none of the spectrographs was judged to have any abnormal characteristics that would be indicative of dysphonia.

Ackerlund (1993) described the use of the phonetogram to measure changes in voice quality. The phonetogram measurements showed that, after therapy, the female patients ($n = 22$) achieved a higher mean sound level and retained essentially the same mean fundamental frequency, in comparison to their pre-treatment assessments. The male patients ($n = 11$) did not achieve higher mean sound levels after therapy, but did record higher mean fundamental frequencies. Rontal et al. (1975) provided some individual examples of applications of spectrography to assess vocal change. Spectrograms made at different stages of therapy treatment in a patient with vocal nodules showed a change from irregular periodicity striations and a poorly defined formant structure to more 'normal'-looking spectral features. Also, a patient with dysphonia plica ventricularis demonstrated extreme breathy voice, and the accompanying spectrogram provided evidence of high-frequency energy and a poorly defined formant structure. After a full course of voice therapy (not specified), the patient's voice spectrogram showed no evidence of high-frequency noise and demonstrated a clearly defined formant structure.

These studies have used an instrumental measure to provide information about voice change. However, measuring voice change over time may not be the same as measuring voice therapy effectiveness. An efficacy study that selects one assessment technique in isolation and/or does not relate the choice to the aims of the treatment is susceptible to criticisms of validity. There are a number of studies that have shown a good correlation between different voice measurements, particularly between instrumental measurements and perceptual voice quality judgements. For example, Hammarberg et al. (1986), Eskenazi et al. (1990), and Wolfe et al. (1991) demonstrate a close correlation between specific acoustic parameters and perceptual voice quality parameters. Measures of voice therapy effectiveness that incorporate a number of related measures are likely to produce results that are more comprehensive, more valid and more convincing.

Clinically relevant effectiveness

Conture and Wolk (1990) suggest that voice therapy effectiveness is closely related to whether or not it was 'successful' for the patient. If a patient presents with a number of voice symptoms that are subsequently resolved or significantly improved, the therapy may be seen to have been effective. In this case, the criteria for measuring treatment efficacy are related to outcomes for the patient, i.e. how their voice sounds or functions. Several research studies in speech and language therapy have stressed the importance of examining successful outcomes of therapy in terms of the overall impact on the client (Kluppel-Vetter, 1985; Bain and Dollaghan, 1991; Enderby, 1992). Many medical and health-related professions are now developing patient-centred efficacy measurements as opposed to clinician-based criteria (Finlay et al., 1992; Aharony and Strasser, 1993; Gupta et al., 1993; Boston, 1994; Jacobson et al., 1999).

The potential discrepancy between what is being measured and what is actually important to the patient is addressed in the concept of 'clinically significant change'. Bain and Dollaghan (1991) defined effective treatment as 'treatment resulting in *clinically significant improvement* in the client's performance' [my italics]. This is not synonymous with statistically significant improvement. A measured improvement that is statistically significant may be of little consequence to the client if he or she still complains of the same problem. Similarly, the client may report significant improvement in his or her condition, which cannot be measured by the techniques chosen. Clinical significance is concerned with the overall impact of the level of change for the patient. Assessments of the overall impact of a change are likely to be based on such factors as the importance assigned to the aspect that has changed (relative to other aspects) and the extent to which the change is believed to be a prerequisite to subsequent successful functioning by the patient. A related aspect of overall impact of the change concerns the effect of the change on other areas of the patient's functioning. The treatment effects that impact on the patient's ability to function (i.e. enabling the patient to participate in social functions, enabling the patient to return to work, etc.) are likely to be viewed as more clinically significant than the effects that are limited to one aspect of a patient's voice problem (e.g. levels of acoustic noise in the speech signal).

Determining treatment efficacy therefore requires a clear statement of the goals of treatment. These goals should reflect the problems, needs and expectations of the patient. It is then possible to devise a clear rationale for the choice of measurement techniques in order to determine whether these aims have been achieved or not. The measurement techniques are discussed in Chapter 4.

Chapter 4
Techniques for measuring change in voice over time

Choosing appropriate outcome measures is crucial in the design of a good efficacy study. The wrong and inappropriate choice of outcome measures can invalidate an otherwise well-designed study. Outcomes are multidimensional. Olswang (1998) observes that outcomes are only defined in terms of the agent. Thus, the outcomes can be:

- clinically derived, i.e. clinical measures such as maximum phonation time, ability to sustain phonation, etc.
- functional, i.e. ability to use the telephone, ability to resume teaching job, etc.
- administrative, i.e. number of times seen, client referral patterns, etc.
- financial, i.e. cost of treatment programme
- client defined, i.e. perceived improvement in quality of life.

As we are concerned in this book with effectiveness and not efficiency, we can limit ourselves to considering outcomes that are clinical, functional and patient-centred. Enderby (1992) states that outcome measures are too often related to only one aspect of care, leading to the false impressions of treatment effectiveness. Yet we are still left with a difficult situation with regard to which measurement techniques to choose. There are no established voice outcome packages available and no clear procedures to aid appropriate selection. Furthermore, there are a large number of voice assessment techniques to choose from. Hirano (1989) identified over 50 techniques that were being used for the evaluation of the human voice throughout the world. These techniques can be divided into six broad categories.

Aerodynamic measurements
Subglottal pressure, glottal resistance, glottal efficiency, AC/DC ratio, airflow/intensity ratio, phonation quotient, maximum phonation time, vocal velocity index, pulmonary function test, rib cage and abdominal movements, vital capacity.

Measurements of fundamental frequency (Fo) and intensity (SPL)
Fo range, speaking (or habitual) Fo, intensity range (or sound pressure level, SPL), speaking (or habitual) SPL, Fo SPL profile (phonetogram), vocal register examination.

Visual and auditory perceptual measurements
Laryngeal mirror examination, fibreoptic nasendoscopy, microscopy, stroboscopy, video-stroboscopy, ultra-high-speed photography, auditory perceptual judgement.

Physiological measurements
Electroglottography, photoelectric glottography, ultrasound glottography, laryngography, electromyography.

Acoustic analysis
Sound spectrogram, pitch perturbation, amplitude perturbation, signal-to-noise ratio, harmonic-to-noise ratio, noise energy measurement, spectrum envelope, long-term average spectra, inverse filter technique, voice-onset time.

Other measurements
Radiograph of the larynx, computed tomography (CT) scan of the larynx, magnetic resonance imaging (MRI) scan of the larynx.

Not all of the techniques listed above are, however, useful in measuring voice quality changes over time (a prerequisite for the selection of a measurement technique for a treatment efficacy study). Some techniques are used predominantly to diagnose and determine the extent of the disease and/or condition. Others are used to evaluate the degree and nature of the dysphonia. Only a proportion of the techniques is of use in monitoring voice change over time. Table 4.1 lists the techniques of voice measurement that are commonly used for monitoring voice change over time.

The most common technique used in the published voice therapy efficacy studies was acoustic analysis of the speech waveform (e.g. Rontal et al., 1975; Davis, 1977; Roy and Leeper, 1991; Ackerlund, 1993; Schneider, 1993; Kitzing and Ackerlund, 1993; Yamaguchi et al., 1993;

Table 4.1 Voice measurement techniques commonly used for monitoring voice change

Measurement technique	Aspect of voice measured
Perceptual rating scales (e.g. Darley et al., 1969; Hammarberg et al., 1980; Laver et al., 1981; Hirano, 1981; Wilson, 1987)	Perception of voice quality
Laryngoscopy (Stell, 1987) Fibreoptic nasendoscopy (Welch, 1982) Stroboscopy (Casper et al., 1985; Faure and Muller, 1989)	Visual assessment of laryngeal structure and function
Laryngography (Fourcin, 1974; Abberton et al., 1989) Combined glottography (Murty et al., 1990) EMG (Prosek et al., 1978; Stemple et al., 1980)	Physiological measurement of the laryngeal mechanism
Phonetogram (Komiyama et al., 1984; Gramming et al., 1986) Vocal fundamental frequency (Horii, 1975; Wedin and Ogren, 1982) Spectrographic noise (Emanuel et al., 1973; Kasuya et al., 1986 a, b) Jitter (Wendahl, 1966 a, b; Laver et al., 1992) Shimmer (Wendahl, 1966; Laver et al., 1992) Signal-to-noise ratio (Diaz et al., 1991a) Harmonics-to-noise ratio (Yumoto et al., 1982, 1984)	Acoustic analysis of the speech waveform

Fex et al., 1994; Stemple et al., 1994). Perceptual judgement of voice quality was also commonly used (e.g. Davis, 1977; Horsley, 1982; Andrews et al., 1986; Roy and Leeper, 1991; Schneider, 1993; Fex et al., 1994; Verdolini-Marston et al., 1995). Visual assessment of laryngeal structure and function was used in seven studies (Brewer and McCall, 1974; Toohill, 1975; Drudge and Phillips, 1976; Bloch et al., 1981; Kay, 1982; Koufman and Blalock, 1991; Stemple et al., 1994) and physiological measurement of the laryngeal mechanism in three (Prosek et al., 1978; Stemple et al., 1980; Andrews et al., 1986).

Selecting techniques to measure treatment efficacy

It is important to select measurement techniques according to the nature of the study and not simply on the basis of what is available in the clinic. In general, the selection of measurement techniques should (1) be guided by consideration of comfort for the patient, (2) represent the multi-dimensional nature of voice and (3) match the aims of treatment.

Patient comfort considerations

To monitor voice changes over time, the techniques chosen must be tolerated by the patient on repeated occasions. Ideally, therefore, the techniques should be non-invasive and involve minimal discomfort to the patient. Invasive and uncomfortable techniques have the added complication of being unlikely to measure vocal performance in a 'representative' state because of the presence of the assessment device.

Multi-dimensional measurement

Multiple measurements of a number of aspects of voice provide a more comprehensive method of evaluating voice change, and this is preferable to the use of one technique in isolation. A combination of instrumental and perceptual measurements is more valuable than either one in isolation.

Matching treatment aims

The measurement techniques may be selected to match the aims of treatment. The techniques can then measure the extent to which those aims were achieved. Enderby (1992) states that

> . . . outcome measures must relate directly to the expected changes as a consequence of an intervention. Thus, outcome of contact has to be related to goals, which have generally not been formulated with the precision necessary to permit evaluation. (page 61)

Some possible aims of voice therapy were discussed in Chapter 3. Table 4.2 lists these aims of therapy and the technique(s) that could be used to measure them. This table is not intended as the only way of trying to approach the problem of selecting appropriate outcome measures. It does, however, represent a practical method of attempting to match outcomes to treatment goals. Relating measurements to the aims of treatment helps ensure that the results are 'clinically significant' (Bain and Dollaghan, 1991).

Table 4.2 Some suggested treatment efficacy criteria and accompanying measurement techniques

Treatment aims	Treatment efficacy criteria	Measurement techniques
To restore the patient's voice to normal use and function	The patient reports normal voice use	A patient questionnaire of vocal performance
To improve the quality of sound of the patient's voice to a more acceptable level	The voice sounds within normal limits to trained listeners	Perceptual ratings of voice quality
To maintain the voice improvement over time	No recurrence of voice symptoms within 6 months	Review appointment or telephone contact
To improve the patient's voice function so that laryngeal structure and function are normal	The larynx appears normal to the clinician	Indirect/Fibreoptic laryngoscopy stroboscopy
To improve the patient's voice quality so that the change can be detected by instrumental measurement	The voice shows a movement towards normal characteristics on instrumental measurement	a. Laryngography b. Mean fundamental frequency c. Acoustic analysis of the voice waveform d. Phonetogram

'Objective' versus subjective measurement of voice

There is an ongoing debate in the voice literature about the relative merits of 'objective' and subjective measurements of voice. The term 'objective' is often used synonymously with 'instrumental', with respect to voice measurement techniques. The term 'subjective' is often used synonymously with 'perceptual'. The word 'objective' is placed in quotation marks, because it does not mean objective in the sense of 'exhibiting facts uncoloured by opinions' (Collins, 1991). The 'objective' measures of voice still require interpretation and, in some cases, correlation to other measures in order to be of value. A large number of authors have emphasised the need for objective measures of voice quality in clinical evaluation studies (Johnson, 1983; Perkins, 1985; Fritzell, 1986; Bless, 1991;

Gould and Korovin, 1994; Titze, 1994). The arguments for the preferred use of objective measurement are based on the presumed reliability of instrumental measures, their ability to produce quantitative information and their resolution on repeated measures. Subjective/perceptual measures have been criticised by some authors for being unreliable and reliant on poorly defined descriptive comment.

Reliability

Reliability refers to the consistency of a measuring instrument. A technique with a high degree of reliability is more likely to be of value in measuring change over time. It is generally assumed that instrumental measures of voice quality are more reliable than perceptual measures. However, there are very few reliability studies of voice measurement techniques (e.g. on repeated measures or across different patients) to support this claim.

For example, Morris and Brown (1996) compared the reliability of various automatic techniques for measuring mean speaking fundamental frequency (MSFo). Five male and five female speakers provided oral reading passages for analysis. Each sample was analysed five times by each system. The findings indicated that the three different automatic methods were internally consistent over repeated trials, but showed significant variation across systems.

The same criticism applies to most of the techniques of acoustic analysis. Bough et al. (1996) stated that 'many, if not all of these instruments [*of acoustic analysis*] have not been adequately tested for reliability or consistency' (page 166). Karnell et al. (1995) compared acoustic perturbation measurements from three different analysis systems on 20 patient recordings. The results showed that the frequency and amplitude perturbation measurements were not in agreement across the three systems.

Similarly, there are no reliability data for Laryngograph measurements (Carlson, 1995). Carlson (1995) considers this to be of particular concern because of the observations of factors that may affect the quality of the Laryngograph signal. Electrode placement (Lecluse et al., 1975), skin-electrode resistance (Baken, 1987), fatty neck tissue (Holm, 1971) and vertical larynx changes (Shipp and Izdebski, 1975) may all affect the Laryngograph trace. There have been no studies that have examined the effects of these variables on the reliability of the traces produced by the Lx system.

Not only is there evidence that instrumental measurements are not wholly reliable, but details are emerging about the relative superior reliability of subjective/perceptual judgement. Rabinov et al. (1996) directly compared perceptual and instrumental means of measuring voice quality. They examined the consistency of perceptual ratings of roughness and acoustic measures of jitter. Ten experienced listeners rated 50 voice samples on a visual analogue scale. Rating reliability within and across listeners was compared with the reliability of jitter measures produced by several voice analysis systems. The results showed that listeners agreed as consistently as or better than objective measurements. Interestingly, listeners disagreed in predictable ways, whereas the acoustic measurements differed in a seemingly random fashion. Furthermore, studies of perceptual judgement of voice quality by Kreiman et al. (1993) and de Krom (1994) have resulted in many recommendations to increase the reliability of listeners' judgements. These recommendations are discussed in detail later in this chapter.

Validity

Validity is a matter of whether the measurement technique measures what it is supposed to. The assessment of validity is a subjective judgement.

Content or face validity

Content or face validity requires the examination of the measurement technique in question and a decision about whether it looks as though it is valid. If independent experts in the subject area agree that the test looks as though it does what it is supposed to, then the test is said to have content validity. If a measurement technique has been used in a number of previous studies, then it would appear to have content validity.

Concurrent validity

Concurrent validity compares the test scores with an independent method of testing the same variable. Close comparability between independent measures of the same variable suggest concurrent validity. This aspect may be investigated using correlation techniques.

Some voice therapy efficacy studies have favoured the exclusive use of objective assessment for measuring vocal change (e.g. Cooper, 1974; Ackerlund, 1993 – these studies are reviewed later in this section). However, it is this type of study, which relies entirely on a particular objective assessment, that is most readily criticised for being of limited value in the evaluation of voice therapy. It is often unclear how these measurements are 'clinically significant', how they are related to the stated aims of the treatment or their relevance to the patient's problem. This is a central problem in the measurement of voice in the therapy efficacy studies. The objective measurements may provide quantifiable data, which are seen to be less dependent on subjective interpretation, but the subjective measurements may provide better information about how the patient is functioning or how the dysphonic voice is perceived by the listener.

It would therefore appear that both objective and subjective assess-ments of voice have something to contribute to the measurement of voice change over time. Objective measurements can be used 'to complement the eyes and ears of the examiner' (Fant, 1986). Neither objective nor subjective measurement is as useful in isolation as the combined effect of both. Stemple (1993) stated:

> Objective measures serve as a check and balance to the subjective measures . . . While no single test or single measure permit a total picture of vocal function, the combination of these diagnostic procedures provides a composite picture of how the laryngeal, respiratory, resonatory and psychological systems are working together to produce voice. (page 297)

As all voice quality measurements have limited reliability, the publication of patient data using any voice measurement technique should ideally include inter- and intrasubject reliability data.

Some of the more commonly used and valuable voice measurement techniques are discussed below. Each technique is worthy of more detailed description and this may be accessed through the core refer-ences. Each technique is also critically evaluated with respect to its ability to measure vocal change (i.e. its value in a treatment efficacy study).

Techniques to measure vocal change over time

The patient's opinion

The importance of incorporating the patient's views in the judgements of benefits of treatment has been recognised for some time (see Light and Pillemer, 1984; Enderby, 1992). However, very few voice therapy efficacy studies have addressed the issue in any detail. Llewellyn-Thomas et al. (1984) developed a series of linear analogue self-assessment scales to assess the symptoms and functional abilities of voice-disordered patients. Patients placed a vertical mark on a 10-cm line, which was anchored at each end with a statement such as 'able to speak without any effort' or 'able to speak only with great effort'. Sixteen analogue scales were designed. They were used in the evaluation of voice after radiotherapy and were not, unfortunately, adopted by a study evaluating the effective-ness of voice therapy.

Two voice therapy studies reported patient-rated data in their evalu-ation of treatment outcomes. Bloch et al. (1981) asked all 19 patients in their study to categorise the benefits of therapy into:

(1) 'completely free of symptoms'
(2) symptoms improved' and
(3) no change in symptoms'.

Verdolini-Marston et al. (1995) used a patient rating of 'phonatory effort' to measure the outcomes of voice therapy aimed at the reduction in vocal hyperfunction. However, both of these studies concentrated on rating the severity of aspects of vocal impairment and did not attempt to capture data on the functional impact of the voice disorder.

One recent development, which attempts to measure the functional effects of a voice disorder, is the Voice Handicap Index (VHI) (Jacobson et al., 1999). This index is a 30-item, standardised, self-assessment scale that measures the patient's perception about the impact of the dysphonia on various aspects of routine living. The authors report good internal consistency and good test–re-test reliability. The VHI scores also correlate well with the patient's perceptions of dysphonic severity. Interestingly, a study by Jacobson and Bush (1996) showed that VHI scores did not correlate well with the clinician's judgement of the severity of the voice disorder.

This need for functional self-assessment rating scales is echoed throughout the medical literature. In general, the patient's opinion of treatment outcomes has most commonly been assessed by quality of life questionnaires (Ware, 1993). Some of these questionnaires (the most well known being the SF-36 – Jenkinson et al., 1993) have been extensively validated. However, this type of questionnaire focuses on general well-being and overall functional status, and is not related to any particular physical condition. In the past few years, there has been a developing interest in questionnaires to measure more specific aspects of a particular condition (see Bowling, 1991; Fallowfield, 1995). Consequently, these questionnaires provide more relevant data of treatment outcomes for a specific disorder. However, in most areas of research, there are no standardised questionnaires. Moreover, the more specific the requirements of the questionnaire (i.e. particular questions to evaluate a targeted set of conditions), the less likely that one is available. Unfortunately, there are no standardised patient questionnaires of voice problems.

Carding et al. (1999) describe a patient questionnaire of vocal performance devised to enable the patient to consider aspects of his or her own voice and rate the severity of that aspect with regard to normal voice usage. The reliability of a questionnaire was assessed by a test–re-test analysis (a sample of people scoring the same questionnaire on two separate occasions). Pilot trials also allowed the authors to revise the format or style where necessary and/or delete ambiguous questions.

The validity of the questionnaire was ascertained by discussing the questionnaire with the patients in a pilot study. Patients need to feel that the questions are relevant to their voice problems. There is evidence to suggest that a questionnaire that is irrelevant may be answered haphazardly and may therefore produce invalid results (McDowell and Newell, 1987; Streiner and Norman, 1989). A questionnaire should contain sufficient items to ensure face and content validity.

> At its simplest, this means: does the questionnaire appear on the face of it to be asking relevant questions about the topic of interest? and does the content of the questions cover the area sufficiently? (Fallowfield, 1995, page 78)

There are a number of response formats that may be used in the design of a questionnaire. Llewellyn-Thomas et al. (1984) and Verdolini-Marston et al. (1995) used visual analogue scales (e.g. those requiring a mark on a line between two extreme conditions). The patient questionnaire described by Carding et al. (1999) used continuous judgement scales (also called Guttman scales – Fallowfield, 1995). This format involves the ranking of items in a hierarchy of best to worst, most to least, etc. The patient therefore responds to a particular question with a qualitative judgement – marking the item that agrees most with his or her own opinion. The use of graded answers (e.g. levels of severity) means that the patient's opinion of his or her own voice performance can be quantified and used in a statistical analysis of perceived change over time.

Perceptual rating of voice quality

Gerratt and Kreiman (1993) suggested that the perception of voice quality is the most important measure of outcome from any intervention aimed at improving voice quality. They stated that patients and clinicians decide whether treatment has been successful, based largely on whether the voice sounds better. Unanimous judgement by a group of listeners may provide one of the most convincing measures of the effectiveness of therapy. Despite this, perceptual measures of voice quality have not been highly regarded as research tools in this area. This is because of their potential problems with intra- and inter-judge reliability (e.g. Ludlow, 1981), because they do not provide objective measures (Weismer and Liss, 1991), and because there is no commonly accepted set of perceptual scales used by clinicians (Yumoto et al., 1982).

Perceptual voice quality evaluation requires a listener to judge a voice sample, usually consisting of sustained vowels and/or connected speech, on various parameters such as overall severity, roughness, breathiness, etc. The listener usually rates these voice parameters using one of a number of rating scales (Darley et al., 1969; Hammarberg et al., 1980; Hirano, 1981; Laver et al., 1981; Bassich and Ludlow, 1986;

Wilson, 1987; Eskenazi et al., 1990; Kreiman et al 1990). These perceptual scales often use different terminology to describe a variety of voice quality parameters. Similarly, they often use different types of rating scale format.

There are many factors that may influence perceptual rating consistency, including:

- the choice of voice quality parameters
- the design of the rating scale and
- the choice of the judges.

These factors are discussed in detail below.

The choice of voice quality parameters

The voice quality rating scales that are available use many different perceptual terms.

Researchers have used terms from a mixture of different sources – for example, aesthetic/impressionistic terms (e.g. 'light', 'coarse' – Hammarberg et al., 1986), physiological labels/terms related to laryngeal function (e.g. 'laryngeal tension' – Andrews et al., 1986) and terms related to specific auditory categories (e.g. 'breathiness' – Eskenazi et al., 1990). Therefore, it is difficult to know which voice quality parameters to choose in order to measure voice quality change over time.

Wolfe et al. (1991) reported on the most frequently used terminology in rating scales for disordered voice. They found that the most commonly used terms were also the most reliably judged parameters. 'Breathiness' (usually used to mean audible air escape through the glottis during phonation) and 'strain' (usually used to mean effortful and tense phonation) were commonly used rating scale parameters. Wolfe et al. (1991) reported an 80–95% agreement in the use of these two terms. Hammarberg et al. (1986) and Kreiman et al. (1990) suggest that 'vocal stability' (used in both studies to mean the degree of consistency of both pitch and volume) is also a reliably judged voice quality parameter. Generally speaking, most other parameters (apart from 'breathiness', 'strain' and 'vocal stability') are used less frequently and judged less reliably.

Most authors recommend the use of a small number of perceptual parameters. Wendler et al. (1980), for example, suggested that it was most realistic to start with a minimum number of parameters and used two main parameters only ('breathy' and 'rough'). Hirano (1981) stated that the GRBAS scale, using five parameters, was an attempt to set a minimum standard for voice quality perceptual rating, not a maximum standard. Several recent papers have provided further evidence of the reliability of the GRBAS rating scale (e.g. De Bodt et al., 1997). Eskenazi et al. (1990), Kreiman et al. (1990), Wilson (1987) and Boone (1982) all use perceptual rating scales with between eight and twelve parameters of voice quality.

An impression of overall 'dysphonia severity' or overall 'voice abnormality' has been reported by many authors to be judged reliably (Hammarberg et al., 1986; Kreiman et al., 1990; Wolfe et al., 1991; Dejonckere et al., 1993). Overall severity may be seen as a generic term, which relates to the general impression created by a voice quality (in terms of how 'normal' or 'abnormal' it sounds). Judgements of 'overall severity' have been used to monitor general trends in voice quality changes (e.g. Hammarberg et al., 1986; Wolfe et al., 1991).

The design of the rating scale

Kreiman et al. (1993) distinguished between several different types of voice rating format:

- Categorical ratings: these involve assigning voices to individual categories (e.g. breathy, rough).
- Equal-appearing interval scales: these require the judges to assign a number to a voice sample (where the numbers on the scales are assumed to be equidistant).
- Visual analogue scales: these are undifferentiated lines where the judges indicate the extent of any particular voice quality by marking along the line.
- Direct magnitude estimations: these require the judge to assign a number to a voice sample for the particular voice characteristic being rated. The range of possible numbers is generally not restricted.
- Finally, paired comparison tasks: these require the judge to compare two samples and judge the similarity, relative severity, etc., for each specific dimension.

Most previous studies have used a rating format that is familiar to the chosen listeners and is already tried and tested in that particular clinical setting. Occasionally, the choice of rating scale can also be determined by the purpose of the study. For example, Hammarberg et al. (1980) set out to structure voice characteristics along a complex series of bipolar voice parameters (e.g. unstable–steady, breathy–overtight). For this purpose, they devised a perceptual judgement format using a visual analogue with the extremes of each parameter at either end.

Kreiman et al. (1993), in their review of the literature, observed that most authors use an equal-appearing interval rating scale with a 7-point visual analogue. However, they were unable to find any clear relationship between the type of rating scale used and the degree of inter- and intra-rater reliability.

The choice of judges

There is no evidence in the literature to suggest that there is an optimum number of judges needed to rate voice quality reliably. Of the 57 papers reviewed by Kreiman et al., the number of judges ranged from one judge (Kane and Wellan, 1985) to 461 judges (Wendahl, 1966a, 1966b). However, most (60%) used between three and twelve judges.

Many authors acknowledged the large time commitment required for a panel of judges to rate a large number of voice samples. In practice, most studies were restricted by the availability of the chosen judges, the number of samples that had to be judged, and the number of times the judgements had to be re-rated.

The question about whether the degree of expertise of judges is important to intra- and inter-judge consistency has not been fully addressed. Kreiman et al. (1993) stated that it was reasonable to suppose that an extensively trained panel of judges with a similar background of listener experience would be able to provide the most consistent rating of voice parameters. However, there is no conclusive evidence to support this supposition.

Previous perceptual voice studies have used a variety of types of judge ranging from 'naive listeners' (Montague and Hollien, 1978; Deal and Belcher, 1990) to 'expert raters' (Fritzell et al., 1986; Klatt and Klatt, 1990). Graduate and undergraduate students in speech pathology have also been used on many occasions (Schiavetti et al., 1983; Niebohr et al., 1988). Listener training varied from none (Coleman, 1971), to limited training (Arends et al., 1990) and extensive training (Prosek et al., 1987). The training procedures were often not reported in the studies. For example, Arends et al. (1990) referred only to 'a few sessions' of training and Klich (1982) referred to 'ten minutes orientation'. Even when 'extensive training' was said to have taken place, very few papers detailed the extent of listeners' preparation in terms of hours and content of tuition.

An exception to this was Wolfe et al. (1991), who described the details of two short training sessions. These were approximately 30 min each, separated by one week, and were held before classification of the experimental samples. During the training sessions, the listener practised rating two sets of 13 non-study vowel samples using agreed terminology. After the presentation of each practice set, the listeners compared and discussed their own classification ratings with other listeners. It is likely that judges who have received the same detailed training programme will use similar terms of reference and a similar knowledge base when judging voice quality. It is also assumed that this training will subsequently enhance intra-judge reliability.

Intra- and inter-judge agreement and reliability

Intra-judge agreement is most commonly examined by test–re-test study designs. Kreiman et al. reported that about 70% of the 57 studies that they reviewed had used some form of test–re-test measure. Many of these studies reported satisfactory intra-judge reliability. It is likely that intra- and inter-judge agreement is influenced by a complex interaction of the type of voices being judged, the type of rating scale selected, the type of judges being used (naive/experienced) and how they were trained.

   A review of the literature is therefore able to provide some recommendations to help establish maximum reliability of voice quality ratings. The value of perceptual voice quality judgement as a measure of voice change after treatment may be enhanced if:

- The judges have a similar amount of voice training and experience.
- The voice quality judgements are done by a group of judges with no previous knowledge of the patients in the study.
- The rating scale uses voice quality parameters that are clearly defined and that are fully understood by the judges.
- The inter- and intra-judge reliability is reported. Poor inter- or intra-judge consistency may reduce the value of the perceptual judgement results.

Indirect/fibreoptic laryngoscopy

Visual examination of the larynx may be performed in a variety of different ways. Indirect laryngoscopy involves the examination of the larynx via a mirror placed in the nasopharynx. Light is reflected off the mirror, enabling the examiner to view the larynx (Hirano, 1981). Rigid endoscopy involves the use of a powered light source (built into the endoscope) to provide an illuminated view of the larynx. Both indirect laryngoscopy and rigid endoscopy require oral insertion, and therefore preclude study of laryngeal actions during anything but sustained vowel phonation. In recent years, flexible fibreoptic nasendoscopy has become the preferred technique for some laryngologists (Welch, 1982). The flexible fibreoptic scope is passed transnasally, through the nasopharynx, and sits just above the larynx. This technique allows examination of voice production without impeding lingual function and during connected speech (Havas and Priestley, 1993; Pemberton et al., 1993).

Rigid and fibreoptic endoscopes may also be used in conjunction with a stroboscopic light source (Bless et al., 1987; Bless, 1991). A stroboscopic light source flashes pulses of light in relation to the vibratory speed of the vocal folds during phonation. If these light flashes are slightly asynchronous with the vibratory pattern, the optical illusion is similar to a 'slow motion' viewing of the vocal fold vibration. The advantage of this technique is that it allows careful examination of the laryngeal mucosal waveform during phonation. [In the normal vocal fold, waves travelling on the mucosa from the inferior to its superior surface are observed during vibrations. This wave is called a mucosal wave or a travelling wave on the mucosa. Existence of a soft, pliant, superficial layer of vocal fold tissue is supposed to be essential for the occurrence of the mucosal wave (Hirano and Hartmann, 1986).] Stroboscopic examination of the mucosal wave may have significant value for the early diagnosis of organic laryngeal pathology (Hirano, 1981; Kitzing, 1985; Hirano and Bless, 1993). However, once organic pathology has been excluded, stroboscopy seems to have little value in further characterisation of non-organic dysphonias (Wendler, 1992; Ackerlund, 1993).

If indirect laryngoscopy, rigid endoscopy and fibreoptic endoscopy are not possible, then laryngeal examination under a general anaesthetic may be performed by the laryngologist. Direct laryngoscopy cannot provide any information with regard to laryngeal movement and coordination during phonation.

Visual examination of the larynx has been used in a number of studies of voice therapy efficacy (Brewer and McCall, 1974; Toohill, 1975; Drudge and Phillips, 1976; Bloch et al., 1981; Kay, 1982; Koufman and Blalock, 1991; Stemple et al., 1994). Not surprisingly, most of these studies aim to examine the value of voice therapy in reducing the size of the specific lesions that are assumed to be caused by poor phonatory function. Brewer and McCall (1974) describe some visible laryngeal changes during voice therapy for three patients with 'disturbed laryngeal physiology'. The authors suggest that such information makes possible a more definitive treatment plan. Documentation of progress and comparison to the pre-treatment laryngeal physiology were shown by the authors to be of considerable therapeutic value. The main problem in using visual examination of the larynx to document voice change is the reliance on subjective judgement. In this respect, comments following endoscopic examination are potentially no more reliable or unreliable than auditory perceptual judgements of voice quality.

There have been very few published data on the reliability of laryngoscopic examination. Dikkers and Schutte (1991) compared the written opinions of 38 ENT doctors who visually inspected slides of 45 individual larynges during phonation and breathing. The results showed great variation between clinicians in interpretation and naming of the lesions that presented. There have been no studies of intra- or inter-examiner variation using fibreoptic laryngoscopic examination or comparison with indirect laryngoscopy. Furthermore, visual examination techniques offer little opportunity for empirical measurement. At the present time, stroboscopic images can be either described or judged using a perceptual visual rating scale (e.g. Bless, 1991). McGlashan et al. (1995) describe a system to analyse the three-dimensional image of the vibrating laryngeal waveform by computer. However, this system is in a very early stage of development. Johnson et al. (1996) have successfully measured the glottal area from video-endoscopic images of the larynx, using a computer-assisted analysis package. However, as a result of problems of the fish-eye distortion and the orientation of the scope in relation to the object of interest, these measurements have been calculated only in dimensionless units. Although techniques of visual examination of the larynx remain one of the most common techniques for assessing laryngeal function, they currently provide limited measurement of vocal change over time.

Laryngographic measurement of vocal function

Laryngography (also called electroglottography and electrolaryngography) is a technique that is used to measure aspects of vocal fold contact during voiced phonation (Fabre, 1957; Fourcin , 1974; Fourcin et al., 1995). The Laryngograph operates by sensing the electrical conductance between two electrodes, which are placed superficially, one on either side of the speaker's neck, at the level of the larynx. The Laryngograph monitors the varying electrical conductance between the two electrodes during the vibratory cycle of the vocal folds. Current flow will be at a maximum when the vocal folds are in contact, and at a minimum when they are apart. The output waveform (Lx) can be viewed on an oscilloscope or, more commonly, on a computer interface system, which functions as an oscilloscope.

There is some controversy about the best use of the Lx waveform as a measure of voice quality. Abberton et al. (1989) suggested that the Lx waveform may be of value in the examination of aspects of abnormal vocal function. They described a number of Lx trace patterns in relation to auditory perceptual qualities and laryngeal examination findings. Furthermore, they suggested that the measurements at the opening and closing phases, in particular, may be of value in detecting and quantifying aspects of abnormal laryngeal movement. In contrast, however, Baken (1987) stated that 'quantification of phases of the Lx cycle is of questionable validity' (page 224), because of the very limited information about the open phase of the vocal fold vibratory cycle. With our current level of knowledge, Baken (1987) suggested that it may be best to interpret Lx traces qualitatively. McFarlane and Watterson (1991), in a review of the clinical use of the Laryngograph, stated that although 'a number of measurements can be obtained from [the] traces . . . it may be better to confine interpretations to the overall patterns of traces' (page 113). Therefore, the controversy remains because there is no empirical evidence to support either view. There are no published data on open and closed phase values with respect to dysphonic type or pathological diagnosis (Carlson, 1995). Similarly, there are very limited normative data and the range of normal open and closed phase values is not known.

Several other authors provide examples in which the Lx traces have been 'read' to provide an estimate of normality. Titze (1990) and Motta et al. (1990) have concentrated on interpreting the Lx waveform in relation to expected norms. Titze (1990) described an 'ideal Lx image' of glottal configuration and then illustrated a number of Lx traces that correspond to various theoretical movements of the vocal folds as they make contact during phonation. Motta et al. (1990) attempted to classify the shape of Lx traces and to correlate them with normal, non-organic and organic dysphonia categories.

Fourcin (1981), Kilman (1981), MacCurtain and Fourcin (1982), and Reed (1982) made the following observations about the 'normal', idealised Lx waveform:

- There is a regular pattern to the Lx waveform over time (i.e. each complete cycle's shape is uniform with each corresponding vibration).
- There is an identifiable point of maximum closure for each Lx cycle (i.e. a peak to each cycle).
- There is a steep rising edge which corresponds to the closing phase of the vibratory cycle. The closing phase begins abruptly (i.e. very abrupt decrease in translaryngeal impedance) and has a very short rising time. A rapid and sharply defined closing phase correlates with good vocal tract acoustic excitation and efficient vocal production.
- The closing phase takes less time than the opening phase.
- The falling edge of the trace (the opening phase) is smooth and longer in duration than the closing phase.
- There is usually a trough in the trace, which is essentially constant with time, where there is no contact of the vocal folds along their whole length.

Lx traces can show signs of dysphonia by the absence of normal features. For example, the absence of an identifiable point of maximum closure may indicate poor glottic closure and may illustrate the vocal fold vibratory pattern of a particularly breathy voice quality. This may or may not constitute pathological voice.

Measuring mean speaking fundamental frequency

Abnormal vocal pitch is considered by many authors as an important aspect of dysphonic voice (Stone and Sharf, 1973; Prater and Swift, 1984; Gordon, 1986). It can be unobtrusively measured by one of a number of relatively inexpensive computer voice analysis systems. However, it has not been used to evaluate changes in voice quality over time.

There is some debate in the literature about whether the mean or the modal speaking fundamental frequency should be used (Baken, 1987). Similarly, some authors have highlighted the difference between 'reading speaking fundamental frequency' and 'conversational speaking fundamental frequency' (Hollien and Jackson, 1973; Ramig and Ringuel, 1993). These arguments have not been fully resolved. Most authors have concentrated on mean speaking fundamental frequency of the reading of a standard passage (usually 'The Rainbow' – Fairbanks, 1960).

The measurement of MSFo can be compared with published data of age- and sex-matched normal values. There are a considerable number of normative data of mean speaking fundamental frequency (MSFo) of normal adults. These MSFo norms are based on white American speakers reading 'The Rainbow' passage (Fairbanks, 1960). A range of normal MSFo values is presented in Table 4.3.

Table 4.3 Mean speaking fundamental frequency values: normal subjects

Sex	MSFo (Hz)	Range of means (Hz)
Male (26–79 years)	110–113 (Horii , 1975; Mysak, 1959; Michel, 1968)	84-151 (Horii, 1975 – only data available)
Female (20–50 years)	186–199 (Saxman and Burk, 1967; Hollien and Paul, 1969; Stoicheff, 1981)	168–241 (Saxman and Burk, 1967; Hollien and Paul, 1969; Stoicheff, 1981)

A working definition of 'abnormal' MSFo values may be those that were outside the range of the MSFo values listed above.

Phonetogram

The so-called phonetogram is a graph showing the sound pressure level versus fundamental frequency of voice in soft and loud phonation

(Gramming et al., 1986). The patient is presented with stimulus tones at a number of different graded frequencies and is required to sustain a vowel at a matching vocal pitch. Minimal sustainable intensity is elicited by instructing the patient to say the vowel as softly as possible without whispering; maximal intensity is generated by having him or her shout it as loudly as possible without screaming. Several trials at each frequency and intensity are made. The extreme values for each condition are the data which are plotted on each axis of a graph to determine the vocal 'space' for the patient. Phonetogram measurements have been used to infer laryngeal physiology in several papers (Gramming et al., 1986; Gramming, 1988; Gramming et al., 1991; Ackerlund, 1993). However, these inferences have not been substantiated, and several authors have questioned the reliability of phonetographic measurement (Coleman, 1993; Hacki, 1996). Airainer and Klingholz (1993) and Ackerlund (1993) use phonetogram readings to evaluate changes in non-organic dysphonia patients before and after therapy.

Acoustic analysis of the speech waveform

Acoustic analysis of the speech waveform constitutes one of the most common measures of voice quality change. As a technique it has many advantages; it is unobtrusive, numerical and relatively cheaply available (compared with 10 years ago). However, acoustic analysis is a complicated subject and, like any technique that is applied without a reasonable understanding of how it works, the results can be misleading. The literature on the subject is complicated. There are a large number of different acoustic parameters to measure and a variety of different calculation methods proposed for the same acoustic parameter. There is no standard methodology for capturing or analysing speech samples. There is limited information about the range of normative data for most acoustic parameters. As acoustic analysis has become a significantly powerful instrumental measure of voice change, it would seem to be appropriate to deal with some of the complications here. If the principles of the technique are understood and the limitations acknowledged, then the technique is more likely to be appropriately applied.

Acoustic analysis of the waveform is based on the fact that laryngeal pathology alters the normal vibratory pattern of the vocal folds, and that there is a relationship between the vibratory patterns at the glottal source and certain parameters of the acoustic waveform generated by this vibration.

The glottal source waveform

A voiced sound is simply explained as the sound pressure waveform resulting from the excitation of an acoustic tube (i.e. the vocal tract and lips) by a periodic source (i.e. the vocal folds). This source-filter model (Fant 1960) describes the vibrating vocal folds as the source of a signal, and the vocal tract as a complex filter producing the vocal signal resonances. The speech signal provides a composite picture of both oral articulatory laryngeal components. Acoustic analysis techniques of voice quality need to evaluate the glottal source waveform and to minimise the oral articulatory information. This can be done by using glottal inverse filtering procedures. These procedures assume that the acoustic speech signal represents the product of the glottal resonances, vocal tract resonances and lip radiation characteristics acting on the glottal wave. It is possible to determine the properties of the vocal tract by mathematical analysis (i.e. cepstral analysis). Inverse filtering attempts to determine the effect of the non-laryngeal acoustics and to subtract them from the radiated acoustic signal. This would leave a 'purer' or simpler waveform that is more representative of what the larynx itself produced. Alternatively, information about glottal level sound may be accessed by asking the speaker to minimise supraglottic articulation (i.e. by producing a prolonged vowel sound) (Davis, 1977). The waveform of a speaker who produces a stable and constant vowel sound (usually either /i:/ or /a:/) will diminish supralaryngeal changes and provide acoustic information, which largely relates to activity at the laryngeal level.

The use of acoustic techniques to analyse dysphonic voice has been the subject of considerable attention from researchers in recent years (Johnson, 1985). Most techniques concentrate on measuring either aperiodic noise in the signal (i.e. noise as seen in the spectrogram) or cycle-to-cycle variability in the waveform (perturbation, i.e. 'jitter' and 'shimmer'). These techniques fall into two main categories: those that analyse sustained vowel samples and those that analyse continuous speech (Laver et al., 1992). The analysis of isolated vowels is simpler to process than connected speech. The former does not have to take into account intonational changes, phonetic irregularities, and voiceless and speech pause segments. The analysis of connected speech has to be able to recognise and process these segments appropriately. For this reason, the analysis of connected speech is more likely to produce results with artefactual distortion (Laver et al., 1992). Most of the published techniques appear to favour the analysis of single vowel utterances. There are many different ways of calculating the acoustic parameters within a speech waveform. The most common forms are described below.

Calculating 'noise' in the speech signal

In an ideal, perfectly functioning, phonatory mechanism, the larynx would produce a purely periodic acoustic waveform, i.e., the sound waveform generated by the vibrating vocal folds would be perfectly regular in terms of frequency and amplitude. Voice produced by a speech synthesiser can produce pure, periodic signals (de Krom, 1993). However, during laryngeal phonation, the changes in intralaryngeal muscle tension (which result in momentary mass and elasticity changes) and changes in infraglottal airflow will result in a natural degree of normal aperiodicity or 'noise'. A signal with any deviation from total periodicity will show some noise contamination. Air escape through the glottis is one primary source of noise in the voice signal. The more aperiodic the sound, the more noise there is in the signal. The larger the noise component, the more this reflects diminished regularity of phonatory vibration (Sorenson et al., 1980). Comparisons of pathological and non-pathological voices (as diagnosed by laryngeal examination) have demonstrated greater amounts of noise in the pathological group (Hartmann and Cramon, 1984; Zyski et al., 1984). The identification of this noise in the speech signal is seen by many authors (e.g. Kim et al., 1982; Yumoto et al., 1984; Baken, 1987) as central to the acoustic measurement of dysphonic voice

There are many different techniques that have been devised to measure the noise in the speech signal. Yanagihara (1967a, 1967b) proposed a visual interpretation technique to grade the levels of noise in the sound spectrogram. Yanagihara identified two different types of noise as shown in the spectrogram: (1) irregular spacing of the glottal striations and (2) random 'snow' markings in the high frequencies. Narrow-band spectrograms could be categorised into four types (types I–IV) according to the absence or presence of a variety of spectrographic features. This technique may be used as a visual estimation of noise in the spectrogram of the abnormal voice. Emanuel et al. (1973) quantified the noise in the spectrum by measuring the minimum noise value (in decibels) for each 100-Hz segment from 200 to 8000 Hz. [The voice samples consisted of sustained vowel phonations made at a monitored 75 dB SPL. A portion of the taped vowel was repeatedly scanned by a spectrum analyser with a very narrow bandwidth (3 Hz). The strip-chart output was an amplitude-by-frequency spectrum. From this spectrum, the minimum noise level for each 100-Hz segment from 200 to 8000 Hz was measured.] Other measurement techniques include measurement of the intensity of harmonic peaks (Hiraoka et al., 1984), various measures based on a spectral representation averaged over a long time (Hammarberg et al., 1986) and comparison of the original spectrum with a reconstructed harmonic spectrum (Klingholz, 1987).

Kojima et al. (1979), and later Yumoto et al. (1982), devised a technique that attempted to describe the relationship between the harmonic structure and the inter-harmonic noise. This relationship can best be expressed as a harmonics-to-noise (H/N) ratio. Yumoto et al. (1982) and Yumoto et al. (1984) developed a computer-based procedure to calculate this ratio. A series of discrete Fourier transforms was used to estimate the signal energy at the harmonic frequencies and noise energy between them. A ratio of the acoustic energy of the harmonic components to that of the noise was calculated. A large H/N ratio indicates a predominance of harmonic periodicity in the signal. A small H/N ratio indicates a large noise component and a less well-defined harmonic structure.

The H/N ratio is an analysis of 'noise' in the frequency domain. Similar methods of calculation have been described in the examination of the acoustic signal in the time domain (Laver et al., 1992). These are commonly called signal-to-noise (S/N) ratio methods (Hiraoka et al., 1984; Cox and Krecicka, 1990; Diaz et al., 1991a, 1991b). Thus, in these techniques, 'noise' is defined slightly differently. Here 'noise' is detected in the cycle-to-cycle variation in the waveform. In the S/N ratio, the noise is calculated by measuring the cycle-to-cycle frequency and amplitude values for every point on a real vowel waveform, and then an average is calculated. This averaged waveform value is subtracted at every point in time from the real (noise-contaminated) vocal signal. The remaining value is the isolated noise content level of the real waveform. The S/N ratio is an expression of the amount of noise in relation to the noise in the averaged signal. A large S/N ratio indicates a predominance of periodicity in the waveform; a small one indicates a large noise component in the signal. This S/N ratio measurement is predominantly of value in the measurement of steady vowel phonation (i.e. where the patient is asked to produce a prolonged vowel sound, trying to keep the frequency and amplitude as stable as possible – so as to minimise vocal tract changes, which may influence the speech sound signal).

Despite the different calculation methods, all of the authors mentioned above recognise the value of expressing noise levels in relation to periodic structure, and all have found it a valuable index of the level of dysphonia.

Frequency perturbation

Frequency perturbation (commonly called 'jitter') is defined as the degree of cycle-to-cycle variability of the fundamental frequency. In steady vowel phonation (i.e. with constant pitch and volume), the degree of jitter may also provide an index of the stability of the phonatory mechanism. Jitter is usually concerned with only short-term variation – how much one period differs from the period that immediately follows it. Wendahl (1966a, 1966b) used synthetic stimuli to establish a relationship between random variations in fundamental frequency and perceived harshness. Beckett (1969) demonstrated that this relationship may be caused by vocal constriction. According to Beckett, vocal constriction refers to 'the tightness and/or squeezing in and around the throat that a speaker experiences during phonation' (page 416). He demonstrated that subjects' phonations at increasing degrees of vocal constriction resulted in corresponding increases in jitter measurements. Presumably, increased vocal constriction results in decreased stability of the phonatory mechanism, which in turn leads to an increase in frequency perturbation.

It is clear that jitter is a measurement of some aspects of dysphonic voice. However, it is only one component of the complex acoustic characteristics of a dysphonic waveform. Zyski et al. (1984) demonstrated some degree of discrimination between normal and pathological groups using jitter measurements, but warned that a considerable proportion of the pathological cases was included within the 'normal' range of values. Frequency perturbation seems sensitive to some pathological changes in the phonatory process but, as Hammarberg et al. (1986) point out, it should not be used as a sole diagnostic tool because it accounts for a only portion of what is 'abnormal' in the dysphonic waveform.

It is important to note that there are many different ways of defining frequency perturbation (Laver et al., 1992). Liberman (1961) established the fundamental principle of calculating the variability (in his case – the distribution of the magnitude of the differences) between adjacent periods of the waveform. Since then several variations of perturbation calculation have been proposed (i.e. directional perturbation factor – Hecker and Kreul, 1971; relative average perturbation – Koike 1973; jitter factor – Hollien and Jackson, 1973; frequency perturbation quotient – Takahashi and Koike, 1975; period variability index – Deal and Emanuel, 1978; and jitter ratio – Horii, 1979). Baken (1987) suggests that Fo perturbation measures are likely to be sensitive to phonatory pathologies, although comparison across studies that have used different jitter calculation techniques may be problematic. Zyski et al. (1984) compared all of the most common methods of Fo perturbation calculation. They concluded that there was a similar degree of discrimination between normal and pathological voices by most Fo perturbation measures. However, they did suggest that a study that uses jitter measurements should describe the calculation method used for the purpose of clarity.

Amplitude perturbation

Measurements of amplitude perturbation ('shimmer'), such as frequency perturbation, are also indications of short-term variability in the vocal signal. However, amplitude perturbation is a measurement of the amount of peak amplitude variability from one cycle to the next (Wendahl, 1966a, 1966b; Takahashi and Koike, 1975; Horii, 1980). Similar to his jitter studies, Wendahl (1966a, 1966b) demonstrated that, using synthetic stimuli, there was a close relationship between perceived roughness and measurements of shimmer. Again, in a phonatory task where voice amplitude is intended to be constant, cycle-to-cycle variation may well be indicative of a disordered or inadequate phonatory mechanism. Similar to jitter measurements, there are a number of different calculation methods for shimmer. These include directional perturbation (amplitude) factor (Hecker and Kreul, 1971), amplitude perturbation quotient (Takahashi and Koike, 1975) and amplitude variability index (Deal and Emanuel, 1978). Again, for the sake of clarity, it may be advisable that the use of shimmer measurements should be accompanied by a description of the method of calculation used.

So, it is possible to see that acoustic analysis techniques can be powerful measures of voice quality but that they are plagued with pitfalls. As there is no standardisation of how to collect the data, this procedure should be detailed in the methodology. It is also important to define the acoustic terms and describe the methods of calculation used. As a result of suspicious reliability studies in recent years, it would also be advisable to report one's own reliability data (i.e. test–re-test repeated measures). Finally, acoustic measures should not be used in isolation. They are powerful tools if used in conjunction with other measures, such as auditory perceptual ratings or video-stroboscopic observations.

Conclusions

A variety of measurement techniques is available to evaluate changes in voice quality and voice performance after therapy. These techniques represent a range of perceptual and instrumental techniques. The measurement techniques should be selected to match the therapy aims and should be used to measure whether or not those aims were achieved. Correlations between measurement techniques may provide stronger evidence of voice change over time (i.e. that the voice changed along a number of different parameters). Correlations between techniques may also provide further insight into the interrelationship of different perceptual, physiological and acoustic aspects of voice.

Chapter 5
A clinical study of the effectiveness of voice therapy for patients with non-organic dysphonia

The aim of this study was to evaluate the efficacy of two different programmes of therapy for patients diagnosed as having non-organic dysphonia. This study is published in *The Journal of Voice* (Carding et al., 1999). It has been republished here with more detail because it represents a clinically based approach to documenting the effectiveness of voice therapy treatment. Many of the issues discussed in the previous chapters of this book have been addressed in this study.

Defining 'non-organic dysphonia'

For the purpose of this study, non-organic dysphonia refers to disordered voice when laryngoscopy (including stroboscopy) reveals either (1) no significant organic impairment in terms of laryngeal structure or function or (2) minor laryngeal pathology attributed to excessive voice use and abuse (Van Thal, 1961). In either case, surgical intervention is not considered to be appropriate. Organic and non-organic voice disorders are considered to be on a continuum. Hence, the diagnosis of non-organic dysphonia in this study includes patients with minor inflammatory disorders (i.e. minor laryngeal oedema, non-fibrous nodules, chronic laryngitis) and muscle tension disorders (i.e. supraglottic tension and dysphonia plica ventricularis).

Defining the treatment for non-organic dysphonia

The treatment of non-organic dysphonia does not involve any surgical or medical intervention. The general aim of voice therapy for non-organic voice problems is to minimise or correct the inappropriate use of the voice in order to restore normal phonatory function. However, most clinicians recognise that a non-organic voice problem cannot be treated by simply correcting the physiological defects of the phonatory system. Voice therapy needs to address the psychological aspects of the voice problem as well. In most cases, a voice therapy programme uses a combination of *indirect* and *direct* treatment techniques.

Indirect techniques

Indirect therapy techniques concentrate on managing the contributory and maintenance aspects of the voice problem (such as vocal abuse patterns or poor vocal hygiene). Indirect approaches are based on the assumption that inappropriate phonatory behaviour is a symptom of excessive demands on the voice, abusive behaviours that are detrimental to the voice, personal anxiety and tension levels, and/or a lack of knowledge of healthy voice production. The indirect approach also assumes that the management of these 'precipitating, predisposing and perpetuating factors' (Stemple, 1984) will result in the patient's voice being restored to normal. This approach assumes that the dysphonic patient needs to develop an informed and rational approach to the voice problem. In this way, the patient should be capable of identifying the contributing psychological and social factors in the voice problem. Intervention aims to enable the patient to modify these factors: to decrease or eliminate their effects on the voice and consequently to facilitate improvement of voice quality. Indirect therapy approaches do not involve any work on correcting faulty voice production.

Direct techniques

Direct therapy techniques aim to modify aspects of faulty voice production in order to promote appropriate and efficient voice production. This approach to treatment is based on the assumption that the patient with non-organic dysphonia has adopted incorrect and potentially damaging methods of voice production. The patient learns to modify or replace problematic phonation with a more appropriate pattern of phonation. Some indirect treatment is, of necessity, also incorporated, so it would be misleading to describe direct and indirect modes of intervention as being mutually exclusive. Direct treatment attempts to identify the aspects of phonatory function that are at fault and to enable the patient to correct these aspects.

Most of the published therapy programmes suggest using a combination of both indirect and direct therapy approaches (e.g. Martin and Darnley, 1992; Mueller and Larson, 1992; Morrison and Rammage, 1994). However, within the literature there are reports of successful voice therapy programmes that use only indirect techniques (Fawcus, 1986; Boone and McFarlane, 1988). In the present study, a comparison is made between two programmes of therapy, one that is exclusively indirect and one that involves a combination of direct and indirect techniques (the latter is referred to henceforth as 'direct').

Criteria for determining efficacy

The aims of treatment form the criteria by which the efficacy of the therapy can be judged. These criteria can then be used to help choose the most appropriate measurements to determine whether the treatment has or has not been successful in achieving its aims. The aims and criteria for this study are presented below.

Aim 1

To restore the patient's voice such that he or she reports being able to use it for social and occupational needs.

Efficacy criterion: Treatment may be considered to be effective if the patient reports being able to use his or her voice without the previous difficulties experienced.

Aim 2

To improve the quality of sound of the patient's voice to a more acceptable level.

Efficacy criterion: This goal would be achieved if a group of unbiased listeners judged the voice to have significantly improved to a level that is at or near to a normal rating.

Aim 3

To maintain the voice improvement over time.

Efficacy criterion: Treatment would be considered to be effective if the patient does not have any similar or associated voice problems for at least 6 months after being discharged.

Aim 4

To improve the patient's voice function so that laryngeal structure and function are normal.

Efficacy criterion: This goal can be achieved only in those patients in whom laryngeal structure and function were abnormal at the pre-treatment assessment. Treatment may be considered effective if there are no signs of abnormal phonation at laryngoscopic examination.

Aim 5

To improve the patient's vocal quality so that the change can be detected by instrumental measurement.

Efficacy criterion: Treatment may be considered to be effective if the voice shows a significant positive change on a variety of instrumental measurement techniques after therapy.

Method

Subjects

Forty-five dysphonic patients were recruited for the study. All were diagnosed as having non-organic dysphonia and had been referred to the Department of Speech and Voice Therapy by the otolaryngologists at the Freeman Hospital, Newcastle upon Tyne, England.

The patients also had to fulfil several other criteria in order to be included in the study. This set of patient selection criteria was used to control a series of variables that might otherwise affect treatment outcomes, and include the following:

1. All patients were perceptibly dysphonic at the time of initial assessment (as judged by a senior speech and language therapist).
2. All patients reported that their present voice problem began within the last 12 months. Patients with long-standing dysphonia (e.g. over 12 months) have been reported to be less responsive to voice therapy (Freeman, 1986).
3. Patients were excluded from the study if they reported a history of smoking or a level of alcohol consumption that averaged more than 5 units/day. The effects of smoking and alcohol are known to affect the voice and may affect voice therapy outcomes.
4. Patients with a known psychiatric illness were excluded from the study as were patients with a history of psychosomatic illnesses. Patients with a dominant psychological aspect to their dysphonia may be unresponsive to voice therapy only and may require additional therapeutic input from a clinical psychologist (Butcher et al., 1987).
5. Professional voice users (e.g. actors, singers) were not included in the study. Professional voice users often have excessive demands on

their voice and generally require highly specific or intensive therapy (Sataloff, 1991).

6. Patients were also excluded from the study if they reported experience of previous speech/voice therapy, or had no apparent motivation to change (e.g. expression of no interest in participating in therapy) or were unable to attend regular sessions (e.g. unable to arrange for time off work).

7. Finally, patients with severe hearing loss, needing special consideration, were treated separately.

Treatment groups

All patients were informed of the nature of the study and that they would be allocated to one of three treatment groups and receive a different programme of treatment accordingly. Patients were able to refuse to participate if they so wished, and they were aware that this would not affect their right to voice therapy outwith the study. In fact only one patient declined to enter into the study and he was subsequently treated outside of the project.

The patients were allocated in rotation to one of three treatment groups (T1, T2 and T3). Patients in T1 attended their assessment appointments and were told that they would not receive treatment until 12 weeks had elapsed. It was explained that the aim of assigning patients to this group was to ascertain the extent to which their voice might improve without any active treatment. These patients served as a temporary control group for a total of 12 weeks. Patients in T2 attended for assessments and received a combination of indirect treatments once a week, as considered suitable for each individual patient. Patients in T3 received a weekly programme of direct and indirect treatment with a strong emphasis on direct therapy, but also including appropriate consideration of indirect work. Details of each patient's individual treatment programme can be found in Appendix 5.2a (p.89).

Of the total of 45 patients in the study, 12 were men and 33 were women. The age range was 18–76 years with a mean of 43 years. The composition of patients across treatment groups is shown in Table 5.1.

Study design

The study design is represented in Figure 5.1. All patients were assessed before their treatment programme began. After the treatment period, the patients were assessed a second time and then again at a review one month later. The difference between the first and third assessments was used to measure the degree of change. The second stage assessment

Table 5.1 The composition of patients across treatment groups

Group	Desscription
1	Mean age = 36.6 years (range: 22–68 years)
	Male:female ratio = 3:12
	Mean onset of dysphonia = 17 weeks
	(range: 5–42 weeks)
2	Mean age = 48.7 years (range:18–76 years)
	Male:female ratio = 4:11
	Mean onset of dysphonia = 24 weeks
	(range: 6–48 weeks)
3	Mean age = 45.4 years (range:18–75 years)
	Male:female ratio = 2:13
	Mean onset of dysphonia = 29 weeks
	(range: 5–41 weeks)

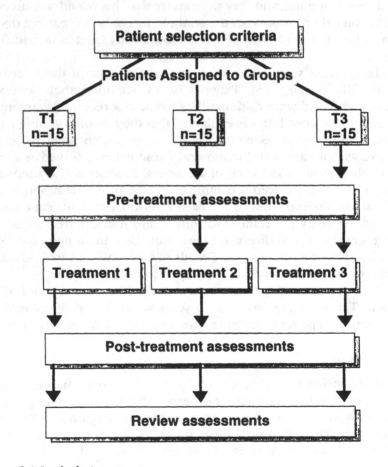

Figure 5.1 Study design

(after treatment and before review) was taken as a precautionary measure in those cases where deterioration may occur after treatment has ceased.

Patients in T1 and T2 who did not improve during the 12-week study period were then offered a course of direct and indirect voice therapy as per T3. The results of the second course of treatment for those patients are reported separately.

Outcome measurements

A series of measurement techniques were used to establish a baseline from which change in voice quality could be measured. The measurement techniques used in this study were selected to match the efficacy criteria and the specific treatment programmes as described above. The chosen assessments are described below.

A patient questionnaire of vocal performance

A questionnaire was designed which enabled patients to consider aspects of their own vocal performance and rate the severity of that aspect with regard to their normal voice usage. The questionnaire is presented in Appendix 5.1. By assigning a numerical value of 1 for every (a) answer, 2 for every (b) answer, etc., a total severity score was calculated for each patient. The range of possible total scores was 12 (normal voice functioning as perceived by the patient) to 60 (severely limited voice functioning).

Auditory voice quality ratings

Each patient was recorded in a sound-proofed room using a stereo tape-deck (Phillips FC 150) and lapel microphone (Sony ECM 144) which was positioned approximately 60 cm from the patient's mouth. Each recording consisted of prolonged /a/ and /i/ vowels (of approximately 5–6 s duration if possible) at a 'comfortable' steady pitch and volume, rote speech (counting 1 to 10, saying the days of the week) and a read passage of approximately 30 s duration (the first paragraph of 'The Rainbow' – Fairbanks, 1960).

Five postgraduate students studying for a postgraduate qualification in speech and language pathology were used as independent judges. They all participated in seven 90-min group training sessions, each separated by a week, before making judgements on the voice samples in this study. During this training, the judges were played various examples of disordered and normal voice samples and they rated them accordingly. Discussion among the students was permitted throughout the training period.

It was originally intended to ask a set of judges to rate all of the voices (pre- and post-therapy) on a detailed rating scale. However, it became clear that this task would be excessively demanding on the judges. Therefore, for practical reasons, the judges rated all 45 patients (pre-treatment and review – 90 voice samples) on an overall severity scale (1 = normal to 7 = very severe). A more detailed perceptual judgement was performed on a selection of patients and these findings are reported elsewhere (Carding and Horsley, 1992).

All of the voice samples were played to the judges via a loudspeaker system. Before the presentation of the study samples, three other voice samples were used as a practice to focus the judges' auditory perceptual skills. The 90 voice samples were randomly presented, so that the judges could have no way of knowing whether the sample was before or after treatment or from which treatment group they had been taken. For each voice sample, the age and sex of the patient were given. No other information about the patients was given and no discussion between judges was allowed during the rating sessions. The 90 voice samples were presented in one session with short breaks of 5 minutes taken at regular intervals. For the purpose of calculating the reliability of the ratings, the whole procedure was repeated on a separate occasion one week later.

Intra- and inter-judge consistencies were examined by comparing the original ratings of all 90 voices with a repeated rating of all voices carried out one week later. The intra-judge rating consistency was analysed by Spearman's Rho for each judge. A value of Spearman's Rho = 1 would represent perfect agreement between the two sets of scores. The results were as follows: Judge 1 Rho: = 0.94; Judge 2 Rho: = 0.92; Judge 3 Rho: = 0.93; Judge 4 Rho: = 0.91; Judge 5 Rho: = 0.87. All of these values are statistically significant at p 0.001. Inter-judge consistency was examined by using Kendall's Coefficient of Concordance, W, to calculate the degree of agreement between the judges on all of the 90 voice samples. Statistical analysis demonstrated an agreement of $W = 0.89, p < 0.05$. In view of this high degree of agreement within and between the judges, the *mean* severity scores across all judges were used in analysis of the results.

Indirect/Fibreoptic laryngoscopy

Indirect or fibreoptic laryngoscopy by the referring laryngologist was performed at each of the three assessment stages to observe movement of the vocal folds during phonation and to identify any particular physical manifestations of vocal hyperfunction. Although the patients were examined by a total of 15 laryngologists, each individual patient was seen by the same laryngologist at all three assessment stages. The written comments after laryngoscopic examination meant that the patients could be categorised according to their most dominant laryngological finding.

Laryngography

A laryngograph (electrolaryngograph) trace was obtained for all patients in the study using standard procedures (Fourcin, 1981; Kilman, 1981). The surface electrodes were placed at an appropriate place on the subject's neck at the level of the larynx, and the patient was asked to prolong an /i/ vowel. The neck electrodes were adjusted in order to attain the clearest Lx signal on the computer screen. A one-second portion of the clearest signal (as judged by the author) of a typical /i/ vowel utterance (at midpitch) was captured and printed out.

As a result of difficulties in the quantification of phases of the Lx cycle (Baken, 1987; McFarlane and Watterson, 1991), the traces were interpreted qualitatively and 'read' to provide an estimate of normality. The traces were rated on a scale of 0–5, with 0 representing normal and 5 a very abnormal Lx trace. The rating was therefore an overall qualitative impression of how the trace compared with the idealised, normal waveform. The scorings were based on expected visual norms as described by a number of authors (e.g. Reed, 1982; McFarlane and Watterson, 1991).

Three independent judges each rated the same random sample of 20 Lx traces. These three judges were all experienced voice clinicians who were familiar with Lx trace interpretation. The 20 Lx traces were also rated by the author. No discussion between the judges was allowed during the rating exercise. The ratings of the three judges showed a high degree of agreement with each other and with the author's scores (Kendall's Coefficient of Concordance $W = 0.83$, $p = <0.05$). Subsequently, the rest of the Lx traces in the study were rated by the author alone.

Fundamental frequency analysis

Mean speaking fundamental frequency (MSFo) was measured from the Lx signal with the patient reading 'The Rainbow' passage (Fairbanks, 1960). The trace was analysed by the extended PCLX software package (Laryngograph Ltd), and first- and second-order distributions (Dx) were calculated. The first-order Dx plot shows the raw data, and the second- and third-order Dx plots show the result of 'smoothing' the data in two stages. This 'smoothing' is, in effect, a filtering process, designed to purge the data of extreme frequency readings. Third-order distribution was not available on the PCLX software package that was used. An MSFo was calculated from the results of the second-order Dx analysis. In the absence of reliable normative MSFo values for British English speakers, the results were compared with the normative values cited by Horii (1975) for American males (mean 112.5 Hz, range of means 84–151 Hz) and by Saxman and Burk (1967) for American females (mean 192.4 Hz, range of means 168–221 Hz). 'Abnormal' MSFo values were defined as those that did not fall within these published normal values.

Acoustic analysis of the speech waveform

Acoustic analysis of voice quality made use of patients' production of a prolonged /i/ vowel (about 5 or 6 seconds) with their best attempt at stable pitch and volume. The vowel /i/ was chosen in order to be consistent with most previous acoustic analysis studies (Hillenbrand et al., 1984; Hillenbrand, 1987; Karnell et al., 1991; Wolfe et al., 1995; Rabinov et al., 1996). The taped /i/ vowel signal was low pass filtered at 10 kHz and sampled at 20 kHz using a Computer Speech Laboratory (Kay Elemetrics). The middle second of the utterance was identified using manually operated cursors and saved to disk. This 1-second sample was then analysed using the AUDED analysis program to extract estimates of signal-to-noise ratio and jitter and shimmer. The AUDED speech waveform analysis system (short for '*AU*Dio *ED*itor') was originally developed at Northwestern University, Chicago Illinois, to facilitate the acquisition, display and editing of audio speech waveforms. The version used in this analysis was the version adapted for the IBM PC, developed at Boston University, Boston Massachusetts (Diaz et al., 1991a, 1991b).

The AUDED analysis of the speech waveform provides a quantification of cycle-to-cycle variations in the speech waveform. There are several steps within the AUDED programme that enable the accurate identification of pitch cycles, thereby providing robust estimates of pitch perturbation:

1. Low pass filtering of the signal (cut-off = 500 Hz). The large number of peaks and zero crossings present within a period can make it extremely difficult to determine the end of a particular period. Low pass filtering effectively smoothes the waveform, making it easier to identify the underlying quasi-periodicity.

2. Defining a frequency range within which the automatic marking of pitch periods will take place. AUDED has default settings for normal male and female frequency ranges. These ranges can be altered if required in order to capture all of the pitch markings in any particular trace.

3. Requesting assistance from the program user when the automated analysis is unable to process any aspect of the waveform. If a portion of a waveform cannot be processed automatically, period markers can be identified manually. This is necessary only occasionally and only for a short section of the waveform. Automatic processing can then resume once this problem section has been dealt with manually.

The automatic processing of the speech signal was then checked for

accuracy. The AUDED manual describes several self-checking procedures, which can easily identify potential errors in the period markings
and can be altered manually.

Once the above signal processing has been completed, AUDED
allows the following acoustic measures to be calculated.

Signal-to-noise ratio

The AUDED system uses the following procedure to calculate statistics of
signal-to-noise (S/N) ratio in a waveform (Diaz et al., 1991a). An average
waveform is calculated from the frequency and amplitude information
from each individual period. The 'noise' in each period is calculated by
subtracting the values of the averaged period waveform from each cycle
on the real signal. The total cumulative difference between the averaged
period and all of the real periods in the speech waveform defines the
amount of noise in the signal. The S/N ratio is an expression of the
amount of noise identified, in comparison to the noise in the averaged
signal. If the total amount of noise calculated is small, the S/N ratio value
will be large. Conversely, a predominance of noise in the waveform will
result in a small S/N ratio value.

Jitter and shimmer

AUDED calculates mean frequency and amplitude perturbation measures
(Diaz et al., 1991a). It defines mean perturbation (in either frequency or
amplitude) as the sum of the absolute values of the differences between
the current and the previous period, divided by the number of periods
minus one.

There were a number of voice samples that had either insufficient or
no acoustic data which could be analysed, i.e. the sample of attempted
voice consisted of entirely aperiodic noise with no signs of periodicity in
the vibration of the vocal folds, or the voice signal did not reach a
duration of one full second. It was important, however, for these
samples to be included in the statistical calculations because they represented some of the more severely dysphonic voices. To calculate the
degree of change for these patients, the unanalysable voice signals were
assigned the value of 'greater than the worst value' recorded in the
whole study across all treatment groups. All of these voices represented
'maximally dysphonic' values in relation to the rest of the values found
in the study. This procedure was also followed for the jitter and shimmer
results, which are presented later.

It was also necessary to consider the reliability of the acoustic
analysis system before analysing the data, as a measure of longitudinal

change. The degree of reliability of the S/N ratio and jitter and shimmer values in this study was examined using a test–re-test procedure (10 voice samples). There was a significant agreement between three repeated analyses of the voice samples ($p = <0.05$). There was also a significant agreement between two operators each analysing the voice samples independently (Kendall's Coefficient of Concordance: $p = <0.05$).

Delivery of therapy programme

All therapy interventions were recorded in detail in the clinical notes. The author was the only therapist involved in the treatment of all patients. It was ensured that patients from the T2 and T3 groups were given approximately the same amount of therapist–patient contact time (a course of eight weekly therapy sessions – each of 40–45 minutes dura-tion). Patients in group T1 were seen for initial, post-treatment and review assessment sessions only as they were acting as a control group. Although patients in T2 and T3 received either direct or direct with indi-rect therapy, respectively, the specifics of each treatment programme were tailored to meet the needs of each individual patient. The particular choice of techniques, their order and the length of time spent at each stage were dependent on the nature of the patient's dysphonia and the patient's response to any particular treatment strategy. Details of each patient's individual therapy programme for the two treatment groups were documented in the notes.

Data analysis

None of the data for any of the measurement techniques demonstrated normal distribution at the pre-treatment, review or difference (review minus pre-treatment) stages. Therefore, it seemed reasonable to make no assumptions about the homogeneity of variance of the population distri-bution. A series of non-parametric tests was therefore applied to the study data. A critical level of significance of $p = <0.05$ was used in all statistical tests. These tests are briefly described below.

The Kruskal-Wallis one-way analysis of variance

The Kruskal-Wallis One-way Analysis of Variance (Bradley, 1968) was used to compare the three sets of results of T1, T2 and T3. In most cases, the difference score was used for each patient in each group. The difference score represented the degree of change (either improvement or deterio-ration) between the pre-treatment and the review assessments. The Kruskal-Wallis test examines whether the three sets of scores came from the same population or from different ones. This procedure also uses a correction for tied values (Leach, 1979) – this is important because some of the measurement data involved a considerable number of tied values. With three samples of 15 patients, the critical value of K at the 0.05 probability level is 5.99. Therefore a K value larger than this shows a significant difference between the three treatment groups.

The Mann–Whitney test

The Mann–Whitney test (Leach, 1979) was used to analyse the difference scores of any two sets of data. This test is sometimes referred to as the Wilcoxon ranked sum analysis, and it uses the same calculation method. The Mann–Whitney test was used to examine the results of any two treatment groups for each particular measurement technique. The test examines whether two sets of scores come from the same population or two different populations. This test was used to examine the differences between T1 versus T2, T2 versus T3 and T3 versus T1. The Mann-Whitney test was able to demonstrate which two sets of data showed the largest difference. With 15 patients in T1 and 15 in T2, the tabulated critical value at the 0.05 probability level (two-tailed) is 97. Values *below* this figure are statistically significant.

Results

The data for all patients at pre-treatment and review stages for all measurements are presented in Appendix 5.2. The graphic representation of the difference scores for all patients in all three treatment groups is shown in the report for each separate measurement technique, unless otherwise stated.

The patient questionnaire of vocal performance

A summary of the difference scores is represented in Figure 5.2.

There was a statistically significant difference between the groups' difference scores (Kruskal-Wallis K = 10.91 (after correction for ties), $p < 0.05$ (two-tailed).

Further analysis, comparing the patients' difference scores in one group with those in each of the other groups, showed that there was a significant difference (p = <0.05) between the scores of all three groups (Mann-Whitney test: T1 vs T2 = 70.0, T1 vs T3 =34.50, T2 vs T3 = 56.50). The largest difference in scores was between T1 and T3. This is demonstrated in Figure 5.2.

The results of the patient questionnaire of vocal performance suggest that patients in T3 perceived their voices to have improved the most. [We refer to 'improvement' of voice quality in this section on the basis that subjects were specifically asked to comment on whether or

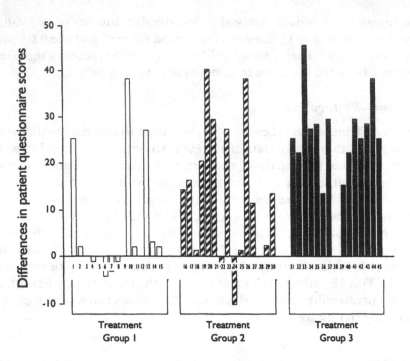

Figure 5.2 Patient questionnaire of vocal performance difference scores for all patients

not they perceived their voice to have improved. In later parts of the Results, 'improvement' or 'improved' is used where change has taken place to make the voice closer to normal on a particular parameter.] This is particularly true in comparison to patients in T1, where only three patients considered their voices to have improved. Patients in T2 showed a variable response to the treatment programme.

Auditory voice quality ratings

Mean overall severity judgement difference scores for all patients in all three treatment groups is illustrated in Figure 5.3.

There was a statistically significant difference between the difference scores in the three treatment groups (Kruskal-Wallis $K = 13.06$ after correction for ties, $p = <0.05$). The largest improvement was between T1 and T3 (Mann-Whitney U = 30.5, $p = <0.05$). There was also a significant difference between patient scores in T2 versus T3 (U = 55.5) and between T1 versus T2 (U = 77.0, $p <0.05$).

The results suggest that the panel of expert listeners judged the overall voice severity of patients in T3 to have improved the most. This is particularly true in comparison to patients in T1, where only three patients were judged to have improved during the study period. Patients

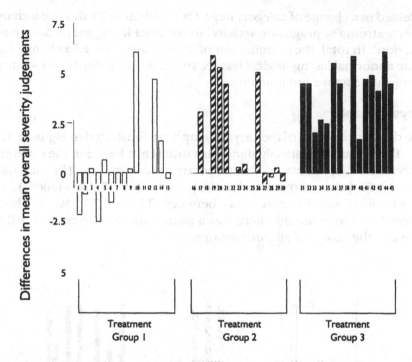

Figure 5.3 Mean overall severity ratings diffference scores for all patients

in T2 showed a variable response to the treatment programme. Almost half (7 of 15) of the patients in T1 and three patients in T2 were judged to have deteriorated during the study period. Interestingly, the three patients in T2 (numbers 27, 28 and 30) had not perceived their own vocal performance to have deteriorated at all (as measured by the vocal performance questionnaire). Correlations between measurement techniques are described later.

Indirect laryngoscopy

The comments arising from laryngoscopic examination were categorised according to their most dominant laryngological feature. The distribution of patients in each category can be found in Appendix 5. Twelve patients in T3 showed a decrease in dominant abnormal laryngological features in all categories, and a subsequent increase in indirect examinations where no abnormality was found. Three patients in T2 showed a change from abnormal laryngeal features to normal laryngeal function. Most patients in T2 remained in the same category as at their pre-treatment assessment – including the four patients who had no abnormality detected at the pre-treatment stage. Three of these patients responded positively to indirect therapy (as measured by the other techniques), but this cannot be reflected in a change of category here. One patient in T1 showed a change from 'extreme supraglottic activity' to 'normal laryngeal structure and function'. In total, the examination of 18 patients showed a change from some abnormal laryngological feature to 'no abnormality found – normal laryngeal structure and function'.

Laryngography

The difference scores of the Laryngograph are illustrated in Figure 5.4.

There was a statistically significant difference between the difference scores for all patients in the three treatment groups (Kruskal-Wallis K = 13.52 [after correction for ties], p = < 0.05 (two-tailed)). The largest difference in scores was between T1 and T3 (Mann-Whitney scores U = 26), although there was a significant difference (p = <0.05) between the scores of all three groups.

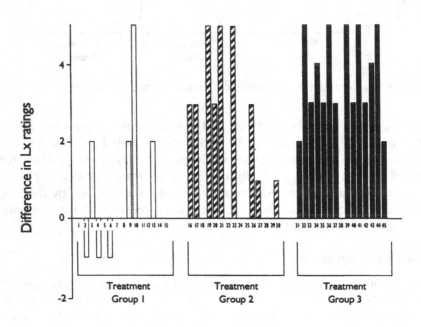

Figure 5.4 Laryngograph ratings: difference scores for all patients

Mean speaking fundamental frequency

The second-order *Fo* distribution values were used to measure changes in MSFo in all patients in the three treatment groups. The change in MSFo measurements for each patient from pre-treatment to review is shown in Figures 5.5 (females) and 5.6 (males). These figures may be summarised

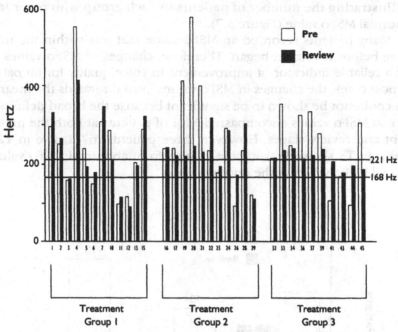

Figure 5.5 MSFo: pre and review scores; female patients (normal female range of MSFo = 168–221 Hz)

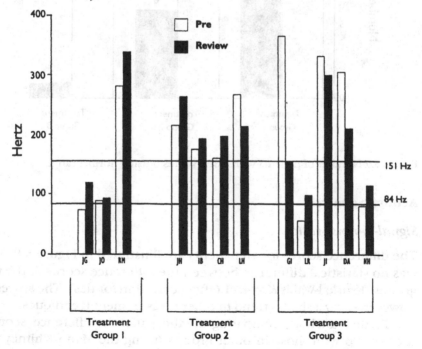

Figure 5.6 MSFo: pre and review scores; male patients (normal male range of MSFo = 84–151 Hz)

by illustrating the number of patients in each group who recorded an abnormal MSFo value (Figure 5.7).

Many patients recorded an MSFo value that was within the normal range before treatment began. Therefore, changes in MSFo values were not a reliable indicator of improvement in voice quality for all patients. In most cases, the changes in MSFo values moved towards the mean, but this could not be shown to be significant because the broad definition of normal MSFo values encompassed a lot of patients at both the pre-treatment and review stages. However, three patients in T1, five in T2 and eleven in T3 showed favourable change from abnormal MSFo values to normal MSFo values at the review stage.

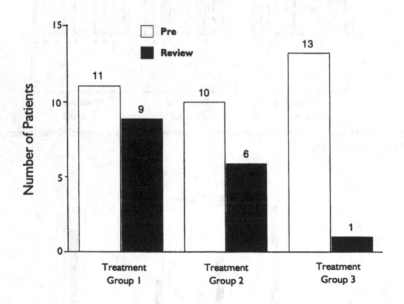

Figure 5.7 Number of patients with MSFo values outside normal range

Acoustic analysis

Signal-to-noise ratio

The difference scores for all patients are illustrated in Figure 5.8. There was no statistical difference between the difference scores in the three groups (Kruskal-Wallis $K = 4.71$ (after correction for ties). The scores did, however, show a similar trend to other measurement techniques.

Further analysis, comparing all the patient's difference scores in each group with those in other groups (using the Mann-Whitney test), showed that the largest difference scores was that between T1 and T3

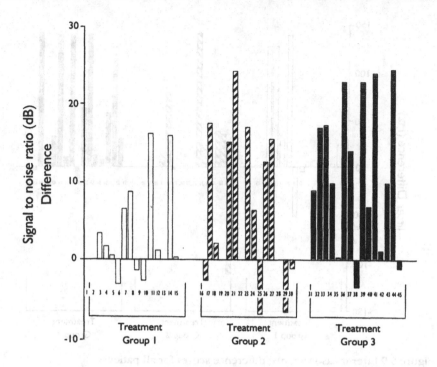

Figure 5.8 Signal to noise ratio measurements; difference for all patients

(Mann-Whitney U= 43, *p* =<0.05). There was also a significant differ-ence between the scores of T2 and T3 (U = 91, p = <0.05) and also between T1 and T2 (U = 93, p = <0.05).

Jitter and shimmer

The difference scores between the pre-treatment and review jitter meas-urements for all patients are illustrated in Figure 5.9.

The difference between the scores in the three treatment groups was not statistically significant at p = <0.05 (Kruskal-Wallis K = 4.47). However, as with the S/N ratio results, the scores showed a similar trend of response to therapy as indicated by the other measurement techniques. Further analysis showed that the only significant difference was between T1 and T3 (Mann-Whitney U = 57, p = <0.05). There was no significant difference between the scores of T2 and T3 (U = 100.5) or between those of T1 and T2 (U = 103.5) at p = <0.05 level.

Figure 5.10 illustrates all patient changes from the pre-treatment to review in shimmer measurements.

The difference between the scores for patients in the three groups was statistically significant at *p* = <0.05 (K = 6.46). Further analysis

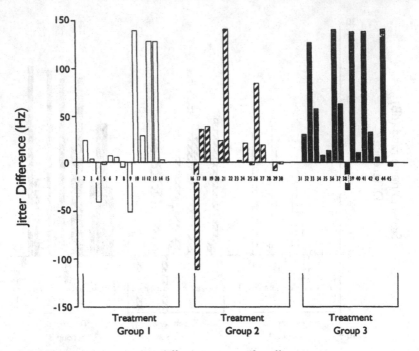

Figure 5.9 Jitter measurements; difference scores for all patients

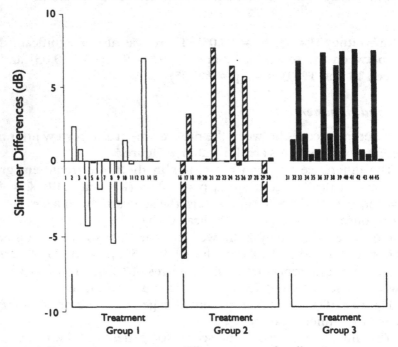

Figure 5.10 Shimmer measurements; difference scores for all patients

showed that the largest difference was between T1 and T3 (Mann-Whitney $U = 57$, $p = <0.05$). This is demonstrated in Figure 5.10. However, for shimmer values, both T1 versus T2 ($U = 107$) and T2 versus T3 ($U = 99.5$) were not significant.

Telephone/review contact at 6 months after treatment

From the original study of 45 patients, most of the measurement techniques identified that 24 patients improved between their pre-treatment and review assessments. These patients were all contacted 6 months after therapy discharge to ascertain whether they had had any further episodes of dysphonia. Three patients had suffered further episodes of dysphonia within 6 months after the completion of their treatment programme. These were patients 10 (T1), 26 (T2) and 33 (T3). These patients all returned to the ENT Department for further examination and treatment. The other 21 patients have reported no further voice problems since their discharge from the study. This would suggest that, in a large number of cases, the benefits of the therapy were maintained.

Correlations between different measurement techniques

The patient questionnaire and mean severity ratings

There was a statistically significant correlation (Spearman's $= 0.648$, $p = <0.05$) between the patient questionnaire of vocal performance and the mean severity ratings. This would suggest that there is a relationship between how severe the voice is judged by trained listeners and how much of a problem it is for the patient. This finding may not be particularly surprising, but it is valuable with respect to evaluating the patient questionnaire of vocal performance, because it was a newly devised measurement technique for this study. A clear correlation between the questionnaire results and the judgement of voice severity by five independent judges suggests a link between these two different voice outcome measures. From these results, it would appear that the patient questionnaire is a valuable measure of voice change and a reliable indicator of voice change after therapy.

Correlations between acoustic measurements

The correlations between the three acoustic measurements are presented in Table 5.2. There is a high correlation between the measurement values of different characteristics of the acoustic signal.

Table 5.2 Correlations between the three acoustic measures

Measure	Spearman ρ_x	Statistical significance
S/N ratio and jitter	0.838	$p<0.05$
S/N ratio and jitter	0.676	$p<0.05$
Shimmer and jitter	0.693	$p<0.05$

S/N ratio and mean severity ratings

Within the literature, reported findings suggest that there is a significant correlation between overall judgement of voice severity and measurements of noise in the acoustic signal (Eskenazi et al., 1990; Wolfe et al., 1991; Kreiman et al., 1993). The correlation between the mean severity ratings and S/N ratio values in this study was 0.529 (p = <0.05). This correlation is of a similar order to that in previous studies in this area.

Further results on unsuccessful patients in T1 and T2

Twenty patients from T1 and T2 showed little or no improvement on a number of tests after their treatment period. These patients were subsequently offered a full programme of direct with indirect therapy. Of these 20 patients, only 10 patients went on to receive the treatment. Nine of the patients either failed to attend any further treatment sessions or declined any further participation in the study. One patient died of unrelated causes.

As all of the patients had shown little or no improvement during their first period of therapy, their final review score was used as the starting point of their second phase of treatment. Each patient received a course of direct with indirect voice therapy for a period of 8 weeks and was reviewed 1 month later. The scores for each patient at the beginning and review assessments are presented in Appendix 5.3 (Appendix 6 in Carding et al., 1999). There was a statistically significant change (p = <0.05) in this group of 10 patients after treatment for the patient questionnaire, overall severity judgements, laryngograph, S/N ratio, and jitter and shimmer measurements, such that for each measure the voice could be said to have improved.

Evidence of treatment efficacy

Patients who were assigned to T3 (for a programme of direct/indirect therapy) showed the greatest change from their pre-treatment state. All of the measures showed a difference in 14 of 15 patients in this group. Four measures (the patient questionnaire of vocal performance, perceptual judgement of overall severity, laryngograph ratings and shimmer measurements) showed statistically significant changes (p = <0.05) after the therapy programme in patients in T3, in comparison to the other groups. The values from the other measurements (MSFo, S/N ratio and jitter) indicated a similar trend of voice change but were not significant at the p = <0.05 level. In addition, nine of the ten patients who had originally failed to display change in response to indirect therapy only, and who subsequently underwent a programme of direct and indirect treatment, had significant voice changes after this second phase of therapy. In total, therefore, 25 patients received a combination of direct and indirect treatment, of whom 23 (92%) made significant improvement in at least some of the measures employed in this study.

The voice changes in T3 may be compared with patients in T1 (the no-treatment/control group). Thirteen patients in T1 showed no positive change over the 8-week assessment period. There was some evidence that several patients deteriorated during the no-treatment period. However, this is based on the results of a particular measurement technique and was not apparent across all or most of the measurements.

Two patients in T1 demonstrated voice change in a positive direction without intervention. It is acknowledged that spontaneous recovery may happen in patients with non-organic dysphonia (Aronson, 1985; Morrison and Rammage, 1994). This is often taken as evidence that many of these patients have a dominant psychological aspect to their voice disorder. In such cases, full recovery is likely to be rapid. This may explain the spontaneous improvement of these two T1 patients, although there was no evidence of any psychiatric complications at the point of screening.

Patients who received indirect therapy alone (treatment group 2) demonstrated a variety of responses. Some patients in this group showed considerable voice change (e.g. patients 20, 21, 23 and 26), some no change at all (e.g. patients 18, 28 and 29) and some, at least on some measurements, showed deterioration (e.g. patients 24 and 25). From the results from this study, indirect voice therapy appears to have been effective for some people and not for others.

There was one patient in this study (1.1%) who did not improve after a course of direct and indirect therapy. Previous studies have reported patients who have not improved after therapy (e.g. Horsley, 1982; Bridger and Epstein, 1983; Roy and Leeper, 1991). Most of these studies suggest that patients who do not respond to speech therapy may respond to cognitive–behavioural therapy (Butcher and Elias, 1983). This patient declined referral to a clinical psychologist and discharged himself from therapy.

One of the aims of voice therapy for patients in this study was to facilitate permanent voice improvement. Therefore, one of the most important measures of treatment efficacy may be the relapse rate of patients once they had been discharged from regular voice therapy. Three patients reported to have suffered further voice problems within the 6-month follow-up time (out of a possible 24 patients who had improved significantly between pre- and post-treatment scores). One of these three patients was in treatment group 1, and cannot therefore be considered as an example of relapse after treatment. The two patients who did have further dysphonic episodes represent a relapse rate of 8.3%.

Appendix 5.1:

Patient questionnaire of vocal performance

1. How do you think your voice sounds now (compared with before your voice problems started)?
    (a) No different from usual voice
    (b) Only slightly different from usual voice
    (c) Quite different from usual voice
    (d) Very different from usual voice
    (e) Totally different from usual voice

2. Does your voice give you any physical discomfort when you talk?
    (a) No discomfort
    (b) Slight discomfort
    (c) Moderate discomfort
    (d) A lot of discomfort
    (e) Severe discomfort

3. Does your voice get worse as you talk?
    (a) Not at all – it stays the same
    (b) Occasionally when I talk
    (c) Often gets worse when I talk
    (d) Often gets a lot worse when I talk
    (e) Always gets a lot worse when I talk

4. Do you find it an effort to talk?
    (a) No effort at all
    (b) Slight effort sometimes (i.e. at the end of the day or when talking loudly, etc.)
    (c) Quite an effort sometimes
    (d) An effort most of the time
    (e) A constant effort to talk

5. How much are you using your voice at present?
    (a) As much as I usually would
    (b) A little less than I usually would
    (c) Somewhat less than usual
    (d) A lot less than usual
    (e) Hardly at all

6. Does your voice problem stop you from doing anything that you would otherwise normally do?
    (a) Doesn't stop me doing anything that involves me using my voice
    (b) Stops me doing a few things that involve using my voice
    (c) Stops me doing a lot of things that involve using my voice
    (d) Stops me doing most things that involve using my voice
    (e) I can hardly do anything that involves me using my voice

7.   In your opinion do you think that your voice is ever difficult to hear or under-
        stand?
        (a)   Not at all
        (b)   A little difficult
        (c)   Quite difficult
        (d)   Very difficult
        (e)   Extremely difficult

8.   Do OTHER people (e.g. close family) ever comment that your voice is difficult
        to hear or understand?
        (a)   No comments
        (b)   Occasional comments
        (c)   Quite often there are comments
        (d)   Frequent comments
        (e)   Very frequent comments

9.   Since your voice problem started has your voice...?
        (a)   Improved a lot
        (b)   Improved a little
        (c)   Not improved at all
        (d)   Deteriorated a little
        (e)   Deteriorated a lot

10.   Since your voice problem started have OTHER people (e.g. close family)
        commented that your voice has improved?
        (a)   Other people say that my voice has improved a lot
        (b)   Other people say that my voice has improved a little
        (c)   Other people say that my voice has not improved at all
        (d)   Other people say that my voice has got a little worse
        (e)   Other people say that my voice has got a lot worse

11.   Would you say that the sound of your voice was...
        (a)   Normal
        (b)   Not quite normal
        (c)   Mildly abnormal
        (d)   Quite abnormal
        (e)   Very abnormal

12.   How much do you worry about your voice problem now?
        (a)   Not at all
        (b)   Hardly at all
        (c)   Quite a lot
        (d)   A good deal
        (e)   Almost all of the time

Appendix 5.2a

Patient questionnaire of vocal performance – scores for all patients at pre-treatment and review assessment (possible range of scores 12–60)

	Treatment group 1				Treatment group 2				Treatment group 3		
Patient	Pre-	Review	Difference	Patient	Pre-	Review	Difference	Patient	Pre-	Review	Difference
1	48	23	25	16	32	18	14	31	41	16	25
2	45	43	2	17	28	12	16	32	34	12	22
3	33	33	0	18	50	49	1	33	59	14	45
4	37	38	-1	19	37	17	20	34	40	13	27
5	38	38	0	20	54	14	40	35	40	12	28
6	35	39	-4	21	45	16	29	36	29	16	13
7	34	37	-3	22	36	38	-2	37	52	23	29
8	37	36	1	23	51	24	27	38	54	54	0
9	38	38	0	24	31	41	-10	39	30	15	15
10	52	14	38	25	50	49	1	40	38	16	22
11	42	40	2	26	52	14	38	41	42	13	29
12	50	50	0	27	28	17	11	42	39	14	25
13	41	14	27	28	54	54	0	43	46	18	28
14	40	37	3	29	39	37	2	44	50	12	38
15	50	48	2	30	49	36	13	45	38	13	25

Appendix 5.2b

Mean overall severity judgements (and range of scores) for all patients at pre-treatment and review assessments

| | Treatment group 1 | | | | Treatment group 2 | | | | Treatment group 3 | | |
Patient	Pre-	Review	Difference	Patient	Pre-	Review	Difference	Patient	Pre-	Review	Difference
1	4.8 (4–6)	6.8 (6–7)	−2.0	16	4.8 (4–6)	4.8 (4–5)	0.0	31	5.8 (5–6)	1.4 (1–2)	4.4
2	4.2 (3–5)	5.2 (4–6)	−1.0	17	7.0 (7s)	4.0 (4s)	3.0	32	5.4 (5–6)	1.0 (1s)	4.4
3	3.4 (2–5)	3.2 (3–4)	0.2	18	7.0 (7s)	7.0 (7s)	0.0	33	4.0 (3–4)	2.0 (2s)	2.0
4	4.2 (4–5)	6.6 (6–7)	2.4	19	6.8 (6–7)	1.0 (1s)	5.8	34	4.8 (4–5)	2.2 (2–3)	2.6
5	7.0 (7s)	6.4 (6–7)	0.6	20	7.0 (7s)	1.8 (1–2)	5.2	35	4.2 (4–5)	1.8 (1–2)	2.4
6	4.0 (4s)	5.4 (5–6)	−1.4	21	7.0 (7s)	2.6 (2–3)	4.4	36	7.0 (7s)	1.6 (1–2)	5.4
7	5.8 (5–6)	6.6 (6–7)	−0.8	22	7.0 (7s)	7.0 (7s)	0.0	37	6.6 (6–7)	2.2 (2–3)	4.4
8	2.4 (2–3)	3.0 (2–4)	−0.6	23	5.0 (4–6)	4.8 (4–5)	0.2	38	7.0 (7s)	7.0 (7s)	0.0
9	6.2 (6–7)	6.8 (6–7)	0.6	24	5.4 (5–6)	5.8 (5–6)	0.4	39	6.8 (6–7)	1.0 (1s)	5.8
10	7.0 (7s)	1.0 (1s)	6.0	25	7.0 (7s)	7.0 (7s)	0.0	40	4.0 (3–5)	2.4 (2–4)	1.6
11	6.8 (6–7)	6.8 (6–7)	0.0	26	7.0 (7s)	2.0 (2s)	5.0	41	7.0 (7s)	2.4 (2–3)	4.6
12	7.0 (7s)	7.0 (7s)	0.0	27	5.0 (4–6)	5.8 (4–6)	−0.8	42	6.2 (6–7)	1.4 (1–2)	4.8
13	7.0 (7s)	2.4 (2–3)	4.6	28	6.8 (6–7)	7.0 (7s)	−0.2	43	6.6 (6–7)	2.6 (2–3)	4.0
14	5.8 (5–6)	4.2 (3–5)	1.6	29	5.6 (5–7)	5.4 (5–6)	0.2	44	7.0 (7s)	1.0 (1s)	6.0
15	5.6 (4–7)	5.8 (5–7)	−0.2	30	6.4 (607)	6.8 (6–7)	−0.4	45	6.8 (6–7)	2.4 (2–3)	4.4

Appendix 5.2c

The Laryngograph ratings for all patients at pre-treatment and review assessments (range of scores 0–5)

Treatment group 1				Treatment group 2				Treatment group 3			
Patient	Pre-	Review	Difference	Patient	Pre-	Review	Difference	Patient	Pre-	Review	Difference
1	5	5	0	16	4	1	3	31	2	0	2
2	3	4	-1	17	4	1	3	32	5	0	5
3	4	2	2	18	5	5	0	33	3	0	3
4	4	5	-1	19	5	0	5	34	5	1	4
5	5	5	0	20	3	0	3	35	3	0	3
6	1	2	-1	21	5	0	5	36	5	0	5
7	4	4	0	22	5	5	0	37	3	0	3
8	1	1	0	23	5	0	5	38	5	5	0
9	5	3	2	24	5	5	0	39	5	0	5
10	5	0	5	25	5	5	0	40	3	0	3
11	5	5	0	26	5	2	3	41	5	0	5
12	5	5	0	27	3	2	1	42	4	1	3
13	4	2	2	28	5	5	0	43	4	0	4
14	3	3	0	29	4	4	0	44	5	0	5
15	5	5	0	30	4	3	1	45	3	1	2

Appendix 5.2d

Mean speaking fundamental frequency values.

	Treatment group 1				Treatment group 2				Treatment group 3		
Patient's Sex and age		Pre-	Review	Patient's sex and age		Pre-	Review	Patient's sex and age		Pre-	Review
1	(F)	59	292[a]	330[a]	16	(F)	47	267	240	31	(M)	56	364[a]	156
2	(F)	33	253[a]	263[a]	17	(F)	58	237	220	32	(F)	39	210	212
3	(F)	22	156[a]	160[a]	18	(M)	67	212[a]	261[a]	33	(F)	40	351[a]	232
4	(F)	36	553[a]	468[a]	19	(F)	50	413[a]	218	34	(F)	75	242	238
5	(F)	25	238	191	20	(F)	37	576[a]	244	35	(M)	69	56[a]	97
6	(F)	51	147[a]	177	21	(F)	76	399[a]	228	36	(F)	33	324[a]	210
7	(F)	23	307[a]	347[a]	22	(F)	18	232	317[a]	37	(F)	20	331[a]	220
8	(M)	68	72[a]	118	23	(F)	48	175	192	38	(M)	28	331[a]	298[a]
9	(M)	41	87	91	24	(F)	27	291[a]	284[a]	39	(F)	65	273[a]	235
10	(F)	21	284[a]	208	25	(M)	71	174[a]	191[a]	40	(M)	18	303[a]	120
11	(F)	42	98[a]	113[a]	26	(F)	43	91[a]	170	41	(F)	56	104[a]	201
12	(F)	33	116	88[a]	27	(M)	27	157[a]	195	42	(M)	31	79[a]	113
13	(F)	19	201	194	28	(F)	57	230[a]	302[a]	43	(F)	32	166[a]	175
14	(M)	53	279[a]	338[a]	29	(F)	57	119	110	44	(F)	53	91[a]	195
15	(F)	23	287[a]	321[a]	30	(M)	48	264[a]	212[a]	45	(F)	66	303[a]	185

Female norms (F) = 168–221 Hz (Saxman and Burk, 1967); male norms (M) = 84–151 Hz (Horii, 1975).

[a]Outside normal range.

Appendix 5.2e

Signal-to-noise ratio measurements (in decibels) for all patients at pre-treatment and review assessments.

	Treatment group 1				Treatment group 2				Treatment group 3		
Patient	Pre-	Review	Difference	Patient	Pre-	Review	Difference	Patient	Pre-	Review	Difference
1	>-8.05	>-8.05	0.00	16	-5.29	>-8.05	-2.76	31	-1.40	5.99	7.39
2	1.45	4.79	3.34	17	1.55	18.90	17.35	32	>-8.05	8.90	>+16.95
3	9.55	11.42	1.87	18	5.51	3.51	-2.00	33	-1.51	15.71	17.22
4	-0.25	0.45	0.70	19	>-8.05	>-8.05	0.00	34	3.86	13.78	9.92
5	7.18	4.18	-3.00	20	-0.54	14.38	14.92	35	-3.33	7.02	10.35
6	0.32	6.95	6.63	21	>-8.05	15.98	>+24.03	36	>-8.05	14.87	>+22.92
7	12.17	20.95	8.78	22	>-8.05	>-8.05	0.00	37	-1.19	12.88	14.07
8	-2.04	0.41	2.45	23	-1.88	14.90	16.78	38	4.44	>-8.05	>-3.61
9	-2.16	-4.70	-2.54	24	>-8.05	-1.77	6.28	39	>-8.05	14.87	>+22.92
10	-2.13	14.14	16.27	25	9.29	2.39	-6.90	40	7.61	14.20	6.59
11	-2.02	-0.91	+1.11	26	>-8.05	-4.19	3.86	41	>-8.05	15.89	>+23.94
12	>-8.05	>-8.05	0.00	27	-0.36	14.88	15.24	42	0.63	1.76	1.13
13	>-8.05	7.89	>+18.39	28	>-8.05	>-8.05	0.00	43	4.44	14.35	9.91
14	7.46	7.66	0.20	29	1.90	-4.86	-6.76	44	>-8.05	16.52	>+24.57
15	>-8.05	>-8.05	0.00	30	-0.02	-1.13	-1.11	45	12.55	10.08	-2.47

The voice samples that could not be analysed were a value of 'greater than the worst recorded value in the study'.

Appendix 5.2f

Jitter measurements (in hertz) for all patients at pre-treatment and review assessments.

Patient	Treatment group 1			Patient	Treatment group 2			Patient	Treatment group 3		
	Pre-	Review	Difference		Pre-	Review	Difference		Pre-	Review	Difference
1	>141.22	>141.22	0.00	16	30.15	>141.22	>-111.07	31	31.41	4.55	26.86
2	43.87	21.25	22.62	17	35.39	2.06	33.33	32	>141.22	17.39	>+123.83
3	5.78	3.56	2.22	18	49.39	12.77	36.62	33	58.55	4.52	54.03
4	19.22	59.72	-40.50	19	>141.22	>2.99	>+138.23	34	10.78	4.68	6.10
5	6.75	8.91	-2.16	20	25.56	3.56	22.00	35	13.28	2.51	10.77
6	12.83	6.48	6.35	21	>141.22	1.96	>+139.26	36	>141.22	3.40	>+137.76
7	6.16	2.25	3.91	22	>141.22	>141.22	0.00	37	67.43	7.67	59.76
8	56.82	61.77	-4.95	23	3.22	2.49	0.73	38	22.65	>141.22	>-118.57
9	77.19	128.23	-51.04	24	50.46	30.43	20.03	39	>141.22	5.17	>+136.05
10	141.22	3.02	138.20	25	2.31	4.50	-2.19	40	9.56	1.22	8.34
11	57.77	30.57	27.20	26	>141.22	58.11	83.11	41	>141.22	5.40	>+135.82
12	>141.22	>141.22	0.00	27	26.43	7.82	18.61	42	43.91	14.48	29.43
13	>141.22	13.75	>127.47	28	>141.22	>141.22	0.00	43	7.25	3.29	3.96
14	7.07	0.92	6.15	29	50.43	58.48	-8.05	44	>141.22	2.36	>+138.86
15	>141.22	>141.22	0.00	30	38.33	39.10	-0.77	45	6.87	8.28	-1.41

The voice samples that could not be analysed were a value of 'greater than the worst recorded value in the study'.

Appendix 5.2g

Shimmer measurements (in decibels) for all patients at pre-treatment and review assessments).

Patient	Treatment group 1 Pre-	Review	Difference	Patient	Treatment group 2 Pre-	Review	Difference	Patient	Treatment group 3 Pre-	Review	Difference
1	>7.89	>7.89	0.00	16	1.42	>7.89	>-6.47	31	2.45	1.01	1.44
2	3.13	0.75	2.38	17	3.46	0.21	3.25	32	>7.89	1.19	>+6.70
3	1.17	0.41	0.76	18	2.04	6.54	-4.50	33	2.25	0.48	1.77
4	1.11	5.32	-4.21	19	>7.89	2.99	4.90	34	0.79	0.54	0.25
5	0.71	0.73	-0.02	20	0.64	0.56	0.08	35	1.02	0.29	0.73
6	0.58	2.32	-1.74	21	>7.89	0.20	>+7.69	36	>7.89	0.67	>+7.22
7	0.33	0.26	0.07	22	>7.89	>7.89	0.00	37	2.70	0.93	1.77
8	1.06	6.46	-5.40	23	0.35	0.39	-0.04	38	1.38	>7.89	>-6.51
9	3.49	6.20	-2.71	24	7.89	1.46	6.43	39	>7.89	0.56	>+7.33
10	2.02	0.60	1.42	25	0.46	0.73	-0.27	40	0.48	0.49	-0.01
11	2.05	2.18	-0.13	26	>7.89	2.20	>5.69	41	>7.89	0.38	>+7.51
12	>7.89	>7.89	0.00	27	1.88	0.85	1.03	42	2.69	1.99	0.70
13	>7.89	0.91	>+6.98	28	>7.89	>7.89	0.00	43	0.93	0.52	0.41
14	0.87	0.80	0.07	29	1.96	4.58	-2.62	44	>7.89	0.45	>+7.44
15	>7.89	>7.89	0.00	30	4.35	4.12	0.23	45	0.24	0.24	0.00

The voice samples that could not be analysed were a value of 'greater than the worst recorded value in the study'.

Chapter 6
The future

The need for more controlled studies

In Chapter 2, I discussed the importance of study design in producing robust evidence of treatment effectiveness. It is generally acknowledged that randomised controlled group studies, wherever possible, represent the most powerful method of examining treatment effectiveness. However, this type of study design has rarely been applied to examine voice therapy effectiveness (Wilson et al., 1995).

In Chapter 5, the effectiveness study used a randomized controlled group design to evaluate voice therapy. However, the study was only an evaluation of the efficacy of *one* therapist's voice therapy to treat 45 patients. Even though the therapist used a standard set of voice treatment techniques, it may be argued that the study represents evidence of one person's effectiveness and not voice therapy techniques in general. It may therefore be difficult to generalise the evidence of treatment efficacy to speech/voice therapy practice. The individual qualities of the clinician may be a large potential variable in determining treatment effectiveness. We already know that therapy outcomes can be influenced by the clinician's attitudes and attributes (Silverman, 1977), by the clinician's personality characteristics (Combs et al., 1971), and by the nature of the therapeutic relationship (Crane and Cooper, 1983). Systematic evaluation of the influence of clinician-specific variables can be examined only by the publication of a number of similar controlled group studies. One way would be to evaluate the outcomes of a number of voice therapists using the same set of standard techniques. This would enable the examination of the effect of different clinician–patient relationships on therapy outcomes.

Efficacy or effectiveness research?

Treatment outcome research is always concerned with the difference between efficacy and effectiveness. The difficulty is trying to ensure a methodologically robust study (efficacy) that is also representative of clinical practice (effectiveness). It is likely that most previous studies of voice treatment outcomes intended to demonstrate effectiveness rather than efficacy of treatment. However, in trying to reflect clinical practice accurately, the studies have often been weakly designed (see Chapter 2). The study in Chapter 5 was intended to reflect clinical practice, while also observing the rigours of scientific research wherever possible. The treatment techniques used were all standard techniques used by most speech and language therapists. The patients treated were no different from those found in an average voice clinic environment. The treatment programmes represented normal practice, i.e. 8 weeks of once-weekly therapy. Patients in the no-treatment group would be equivalent to those on an 8-week waiting list. Most of the outcome measures are available in most speech and language therapy clinics, even though they were used in more detail in the effectiveness study.

However, the results can be generalised only to standard clinical practice with caution. As mentioned above, the study represents only one clinician's outcomes. Second, there was an artificial division between indirect and direct treatment programmes. In clinical practice, the therapist would not be confined to adhering so strictly to one particular type of treatment approach. Finally, the use of patient-selection criteria for acceptance into a therapy programme is not common clinical practice. The sample in this study may not therefore represent a standard clinical caseload, so the results may not be generalised to all clinical situations. The use of patient selection criteria was an attempt to control some variables that are known to influence treatment outcomes. However, other variables (i.e. the patient's profession, intelligence or amount of voice use) were not controlled for in any systematic way. It was hoped that their effects were minimised by random assignment of patients across the three treatment groups. Therefore it is clear that the boundaries between efficacy and effectiveness research overlap. Pure efficacy research has little value in voice therapy practice. However, effectiveness research should be designed to maximise the scientific value of the results. It is not possible or desirable for a clinical effectiveness study to control all of the potential variables. However, it is possible and desirable to control some of the major ones in order to evaluate the benefits of treatment systematically.

Determining the effect of therapy contact time

Without a placebo treatment condition, it is difficult to ascertain the effect of therapy contact time in isolation. In other words, one cannot be sure of the effect of regular contact with a professional who is sympathetic to the problem – irrespective of the nature of the intervention. In all of the previous voice therapy studies discussed in this book, how do we know that the improvement was specifically the result of the treatment and not of other clinician/patient variables? For example, the results of the study in Chapter 5 demonstrated that a combination of direct and indirect therapy contact was more effective than indirect therapy contact alone. However, the study design did not examine the effects of therapy contact time in isolation (i.e. without the therapist engaging in a structured therapy programme at all). The effect of a caring and attentive clinician may be as important to the treatment outcome as the therapy programme (Combs et al., 1971). Andrews and Schmidt (1995) state:

> Both the clinician and the client are partners in the therapeutic process, and it is the quality of the collaboration rather than the skill of the clinician alone that predisposes a successful outcome. (page 261)

The factors that influence the quality of this therapeutic relationship are not well documented. The 'attentiveness' of the clinician (Schmidt and Andrews, 1993; Sorenson, 1992) and his or her ability to be 'precise, friendly, friendly and dominant' (Norton, 1983; Schmidt, 1989) may be important variables in treatment outcome. Norton noted that relaxed clinicians are calm and collected, and perceived by patients as being confident and in control. Haynes and Oratio (1978) suggested that the patient's perception of the clinician's technical skills and empathic genuineness were most important to clinical effectiveness. Characteristics of the patient that may contribute to clinical effectiveness are even less well understood. Andrews and Schmidt (1995) state:

> Despite the undoubted contributions of client characteristics (e.g. personality) to the relational aspects of therapeutic communication, there has been a remarkable dearth of systematic research on the nature and quality of the unique therapeutic relationship forged between each clinician and client. (page 263)

Andrews and Schmidt (1995) attempt to analyse the congruence in personality between clinician and client. They conclude that it was the interaction of clinician/client personality types that was important. Not surprisingly, they also found many permutations of personality factors that are apparent in successful treatment relationships. Interestingly, they also observed that the experienced clinician can and does adapt his or her behaviour in response to the clients – presumably in order to facilitate the best possible therapeutic relationship.

In Chapter 5, an examination of the effect of the clinician–patient contact time would require a placebo treatment condition (e.g. where the patients were seen for regular appointments by the therapist but where no formal treatment took place). It is difficult to conceive of an activity that a clinician and patient could engage in which would avoid aspects of indirect therapy. It would also be ethically difficult to conduct such a study. It is a scientific methodological argument that is not easily solved in the clinical world. In most of the published studies of treatment effectiveness, it remains unclear how much of the therapy effect could be assigned to the regular contact of a caring professional – irrespective of the treatment programme that was being offered.

Dissecting the therapy process

Voice therapy is a complex process. In most cases, it is a series of therapeutic interactions that focus on different aspects of the voice disorder. The progression of the therapy schedule may follow a predetermined structure or change direction according to how well the patient achieves a particular treatment goal. Voice therapy is also often specific to the individual: tailored to meet the needs of the patient. This explains why the treatment programme may differ even for two people with the same voice disorder (Dunnet et al., 1997). There may be many ways of achieving a particular goal with a patient and the therapist's skill is to match the therapy technique to the patient's needs and expectations (and to change direction when the goal is not being achieved). This creates a significant problem for studies of voice therapy effectiveness. Even if a treatment can be shown to be effective, it is difficult to know whether this is because of the cumulative effect of the treatment programme or whether any particular aspect of the treatment programme was responsible for the improvement. For example, the study in Chapter 5 set out to evaluate two different treatment approaches to voice therapy; both contained a variety of therapy techniques. The evidence from the study suggests that both indirect and direct approaches can be effective. However, it does not provide evidence on which aspect of the treatment programme caused or contributed most to the vocal change.

This examination of the cause and effect of individual therapy techniques within the therapy process as a whole is an important area of study. Enderby and Emmerson (1995) identified the need to examine carefully the effects of different elements of the therapeutic process in many areas of speech and language therapy:

> One of the challenges we face is understanding, describing and detailing components of therapy in order to evaluate the most active and desirable features. (page 166)

How and why a therapy programme is designed in a particular way is based on the therapist's assessment and perception of what was required in order to make progress. Detailed assessment may identify a small number of core factors, which need to be addressed (Gordon, 1986; Stemple, 1993). However, how these central factors are addressed may vary from patient to patient. As mentioned earlier, one of the most important skills of clinicians is to adapt their behaviour to complement what they perceive as the patients' needs (Andrews and Schmidt, 1995). How we do this and to what extent are poorly understood. However, it is a subject of considerable interest. A better understanding would not only facilitate more effective therapy (presumably), but also influence the training of clinicians (Schmidt, 1989).

Generally speaking, therapy programmes vary not only in content but also in how they are administered to each individual patient. For example, the decision on how long a patient may stay at any particular stage of the therapy programme is often based on the patient's vocal performance and how he or she is responding to a particular therapy technique. The judgement about whether to remain and consolidate at a specific stage of a therapy programme or to move on is a matter of clinical judgement. It is likely that the clinician uses a complex series of hypothesis-testing strategies in this decision-making process. However, these aspects of voice therapy dynamics are frequently covert. Further research is required into the nature of these covert processes and how they vary with different types of patients. Enderby and Emmerson (1995) refer to this as 'describing and disaggregating aspects of therapy' (page 170). Different starting points and changes in direction in the therapy programme for different people are likely to be the product of a complex therapeutic relationship. Examination of the nature of this relationship and how it influences the course of treatment would be a valuable contribution to the field.

Enhancing treatment effectiveness

Examination of treatment effectiveness is not just a means to an end. The process itself also reveals a number of issues that may further enhance clinical effectiveness. For example, an effectiveness study may show patterns of patient response that may result in better patient selection for therapy. Better patient selection is likely to result in more effective therapy. In particular, the effectiveness study provided valuable insights into treatment selection and patient motivation. Both topics are worthy of further research study.

Patient and treatment selection

For example, in the study in Chapter 5, patients in treatment group 2 responded in a variety of ways to their indirect therapy treatment programmes. Of the patients receiving indirect therapy, 9 of 15 showed a return to normal voicing and 6 did not. There were several common identifiable factors in those patients who were successful: the first was their ability to offer information about their lifestyles and personal stresses and pressures; the second was that each of them accepted that these factors might have a negative influence on their vocal functioning; the third was that they responded positively during the discussion about self-management of these contributing factors. On the whole, these patients were ready to accept responsibility for their voice problem and to monitor and manage their performance accordingly. This would appear to be a prerequisite for a successful indirect voice therapy programme.

By contrast, those patients who did not show improvement found it difficult to identify sources of stress and therefore were unable to accept these as possible influences on vocal performance. As a result, they were not amenable to suggestions of management. They rarely showed insight into their own contribution to the voice problem and could not see the value of self-monitoring and management. For these patients, a course of indirect therapy seemed irrelevant and was therefore very unlikely to succeed. The clinician may attempt to motivate the patient and explain the relevance of the approach, but the treatment also requires considerable cooperation and initiative from the patient. This returns us to the argument by Andrews and Schmidt (1995), who stated that the nature of the therapeutic relationship between the clinician and patient may be central to the therapy outcome.

Whether or not these factors were important in their vocal dysfunction of those patients who did not improve is uncertain. One can hypothesise that the reasons for differences in response would lie mainly with the individual patient's conception of the difficulty. It would appear that not everyone has the ability or willingness to introspectively examine aspects of their lives and discuss them openly. This observation suggests that initial approaches with a patient might profitably examine this aspect. Those individuals who were unresponsive or seemed resistant to an indirect therapy approach would receive direct therapy approaches where the focus was more tangibly placed on correction of inappropriate phonatory behaviour. This would not necessarily rule out the use of indirect therapy techniques at a later stage in the treatment programme.

It is possible that a detailed case history may be able to identify factors that could be relevant to the selection of an appropriate treatment programme. The patient's personality type, life awareness skills, auditory perception skills, etc. may be influential in designing a therapy plan for that individual person's voice problem. A voice treatment programme is more likely to be successful if it matches the patient's expectations of what voice therapy has to offer as well as meeting the patient's needs. This level of psychological analysis of the patient in order to select an appropriate treatment programme may not generally be considered in standard voice therapy practice. It may be that a more careful selection of patients for different treatment approaches may produce further insight into this issue.

Patient motivation as a prognostic factor

A number of questions in the patient questionnaire of vocal performance (see Chapter 5) specifically pertain to issues of the patients' perception of their disability or handicap as a result of their voice disorder. The terms disability and handicap refer to the definitions given by the World Health Organization (1980). *Disability* refers to how the loss or malfunction (of the voice) impacts on daily communication. *Handicap* refers to perceived disadvantages as a result of the disability or severity of the disorder. The particular questions are listed again below:

Question 4: Do you find it an effort to talk? (Disability)

Question 5: How much are you using your voice at present? (Disability)

Question 6: Does your voice problem stop you from doing anything that you would otherwise normally do? (Handicap)

Question 7: In your opinion do you think that your voice is ever difficult to hear or understand? (Disability)

Question 8: Do other people ever comment that your voice is difficult to hear or understand? (Disability)

It would appear from the study in Chapter 5 that patients who scored these questions as severe (i.e. they perceived their voice problem as a significant disability and handicap) responded well to voice therapy. Of the 25 patients who were considered to have benefited significantly from voice therapy, the mean score of questions 4–8 was 4.6 (maximum score = 5). No patient scored below 4.

It is possible to hypothesise that patients who perceive their voice problem to have a significant impact on their daily functioning are likely to cooperate more fully in the therapeutic process. Most speech and language therapists who work with voice-disordered patients are aware of the importance of patient motivation as a prognostic indicator of treatment outcome. Further research into the relationship between perceived disability and handicap with patient motivation may result in the establishment of an important prognostic indicator.

More about outcome measures

Chapter 4 includes a description of a number of techniques to measure voice quality changes after voice therapy. The study described in Chapter 5 used a number of techniques to examine different aspects of vocal function, vocal performance or vocal quality, and how they changed from their baseline after voice therapy. A number of observations can be made.

Multi-dimensional measurement of voice provides evidence of change from a variety of different perspectives

One of the conclusions from Chapter 4 is that, as voice is a multi-dimensional phenomenon, voice change should also be measured from a variety of different perspectives. The use of only one or two techniques to measure change in voice may produce misleading results. It may lead to either an over- or an under-estimation of voice change. This point can be illustrated by Patient 1 (T1) from Chapter 5. This patient perceived her voice to have improved considerably (a pre-treatment to post-treatment difference of 25 points on the Patient Questionnaire of Vocal Performance). However, this change was not supported by any of the other measurement results. There are several possible explanations for this patient's response and one suggestion is her expectation that her voice would improve as a result of attending a voice clinic, even though she attended only for assessment sessions. This may be an example of a placebo effect. Another explanation is that she adapted to her own level of dysphonia over time and did not perceive it as a problem any longer. However, the point remains that taking the patient questionnaire score alone would not provide an accurate outcome this patient.

Similarly, measurement of MSFo in isolation can show results that do not indicate the degree of change for any individual patient. Aberrant pitch levels were not always a feature in all presenting dysphonias. For example, in Chapter 5, a number of patients recorded a pre-treatment MSFo within the normal range even though other measurement techniques indicated that the voice was severely dysphonic. Therefore, for some patients in this study, changes in MSFo alone were not a good indicator of change after treatment.

As there are no empirical measurement tools for voice disorders, it would seem sensible to approach the measurement of voice change from a variety of complementary perspectives. Agreement between patient opinion, auditory perception, visual perception and a number of instrumental techniques (measuring a number of different voice characteristics) provides broader evidence of change.

Reliability of voice quality judgement

Some form of perceptual judgement of voice quality would appear to be necessary in order to measure voice change. A study of voice therapy that omits perceptual voice quality outcome measures is open to criticisms of being invalid. Many investigators (e.g. Eskenazi et al., 1990; Kreiman et al., 1993) have recognised that a rating of *overall voice severity* is the most reliable feature of perceptual voice quality judgement. A rating of overall severity avoids the many difficulties of terminology and rater consistency in the use of more detailed perceptual rating tasks. A good level of inter-rater reliability is the main advantage of using a perceptual judgement of overall voice severity to measure voice change (in comparison to the judgement of individual perceptual features such as 'breathiness' or 'harshness').

The study in Chapter 5 demonstrated an inter-judge consistency of 0.89 ($p = <0.05$) in the judgement of overall voice severity of all 90 voice samples. This level of rater reliability is comparable to the results of other recent studies of perceptual judgement consistency (Kreiman et al., 1993). The intra-rater reliability ranged from 0.99 to 0.94 (mean across the four judges = 0.97) indicating a near-perfect agreement within each judge ($p = <0.001$). With this degree of intra- and inter-rater reliability, the perceptual judgements of overall voice severity can provide robust evidence of voice change over time.

However, the main problem with using an overall severity judgement is the ceiling effect. For example, in the study in Chapter 5, fifteen voice samples were rated as a maximum 7 (i.e. extreme severity) by all five judges at the pre-treatment stage. The ceiling effect may mean that the inter-judge agreement was falsely high. However, it also had the effect of compressing the difference (review – pre-treatment) scores. There was a statistical difference between the three groups despite this artificial compression of the difference scores. Finally, it must be emphasised that detailed voice quality perceptual judgement is still required in order (1) to characterise the individual nature of a patient's dysphonia, and (2) to help plan appropriate voice therapy treatment. Reliability problems may occur when these detailed judgements are used as outcome measures (Carding, 1996).

A good correlation between the patient questionnaire of vocal perform-ance and the auditory judgements of vocal severity enhances the validity of both techniques

In Chapter 5, the severity of the voice quality of each patient (as judged by trained listeners) appears to correlate well with how much of a problem the voice was for the patient (as measured by the Patient Questionnaire of Vocal Performance). It may be argued that a measure of the patient's own opinion is the most important measure in a study of this nature. It is the patient who has identified the problem with his or her voice and who seeks treatment to remedy the problem. In this sense, it is the patient who is best placed to judge the effectiveness of treatment. The patient ques-tionnaire is one way of quantifying the patient's opinion of how their voice problem had affected their communication in everyday life (Enderby and Emmerson, 1995).

The strong correlation between the patient's opinion and the perceptual judgement of voice quality enhances both techniques as valid measures of voice change over time. However, the questionnaire results from Patient 1 (described above) are a reminder that there is not always a clear interrelationship of voice quality, voice handicap and voice disability (Enderby and Emmerson, 1995). The relationship between a patient's perception of his or her voice problem, compared with that judged by others and the subsequent outcome of therapy, needs further investigation. The possible importance of the patient's opinion of voice disability and handicap in determining treatment prognosis was discussed early in this chapter.

Some measurement techniques have a limited role in measuring voice change over time

Several voice measurement techniques provide only limited evidence of voice change. For example, in Chapter 5, the indirect laryngoscopy find-ings were grouped by their most dominant laryngological feature. These groupings were very broad and the differentiation between categories was not easy to define. The categorisation of the patient was based on the description by the laryngologist, the notes and drawings in the medical notes, and, where necessary, discussion with the laryngologist. As a result of the descriptive nature of these data and of the lack of uniformity of ter-minology, statistical analysis was very difficult.

The categorisation of patients was difficult because of the variety of terminology used by the referring laryngologists. Dikkers and Schute

(1991) reported a significant lack of uniformity of clinical diagnosis of benign lesions of the vocal folds between a number of senior laryngologists. Their findings were largely explained by the amount of confusing terminology that was used to describe non-organic or minor organic vocal pathology examples in the study. The results from the study in Chapter 5 further support their findings that indirect laryngoscopy was of limited value for the purpose of measuring vocal change over time. This is not wholly surprising but it is a point worth making because some previous studies have used indirect laryngoscopy as a primary method of assessing vocal change (Bridger and Epstein, 1983; Lancer et al., 1988).

Laryngograph traces can provide excellent information about several aspects of laryngeal vibratory behaviour during phonation. They can provide insights into laryngeal dysfunction and be useful in aiding the explanation of the problem to the patient. Moreover, the Laryngograph is a useful visual feedback tool during therapy. However, the qualitative evaluation of the Laryngograph traces was of limited use in measuring voice change over time. The application of a rating scale of 0–5 in Chapter 5 meant that the system had limited sensitivity. Some traces in the study were rated with the same degree of severity, although they had very different Lx characteristics. Thus, the rating scale interpretation of 0–5 was insensitive to differences between voice types. The small range of values also meant that the calculation of pre- versus post-treatment difference scores resulted in a large number of patients with the same score. This created a problem when non-parametric statistical tests were used to calculate differences between the groups. Non-parametric analysis often requires the data to be ranked before any statistical calculation is possible. Ranking the data in this instance produced many tied values and this is considered to reduce the confidence of the statistical results (Leach, 1979). This therefore meant that, as implemented within the present protocol, qualitative analysis of the Laryngograph Lx signals had a limited role in the evaluation of vocal change.

Acoustic measurement techniques show potential for measuring voice change over time within each individual patient

In Chapter 5, the acoustic analysis results demonstrated similar trends to other techniques in showing voice change within each individual patient. However, these results were only statistically significant for the signal-to-noise (S/N) ratio and not the jitter and shimmer values. There was also a good correlation between the S/N ratio and mean severity rating judgements. Further analysis, not reported in this book (Carding, 1996), suggests correlations between particular acoustic parameters and specific voice quality parameters. This was most apparent for jitter and breathiness, and shimmer and harshness. This finding supports previous literature finds (Eskenazi et al., 1990; Wolfe et al., 1991).

The application of acoustic analysis in Chapter 5 highlighted a number of problems in respect of the methodology and applications of acoustic analysis. These were:

1. How to deal with severely dysphonic voice samples that could not be analysed by the acoustic system.
2. Use of the middle 1 second of the vowel to represent the whole vowel utterance.
3. Use of a steady vowel utterance to represent the general dysphonic quality of the patient's voice (i.e. in conversation).

These problems are now dealt with in more detail in turn.

Unanalysable voice samples

There were thirteen pre-treatment and seven review voice samples that could not be analysed by the acoustic analysis system. For the purposes of statistical analysis, it was decided that these samples should be considered 'maximally dysphonic' and assigned a value of 'greater than the worst analysable voice signal'. Of the thirteen patients who were unable to produce sufficient voice for acoustic analysis, eight improved significantly after the therapy period. It is therefore important that these data are not lost in a study of voice therapy effectiveness.

However, assigning the 'maximally dysphonic' S/N ratio, jitter and shimmer value to all unanalysable voices does not permit discrimination between the severity of these voice samples. This means that acoustic analysis cannot differentiate between patients who were totally aphonic and those who are able to achieve some phonation but not for the required 1-second duration. The difference between total aphonia and aphonia with intermittent phonatory bursts is, however, important both perceptually and in decisions about the clinical management of a patient.

Using the middle second of the vowel sample

It is possible that the middle 1 second of the vowel is not always representative of the whole vowel production. A characteristic of some severely dysphonic voice types is their erratic phonatory behaviour, and it is therefore possible that the middle second does not reflect the overall voice quality of the vowel utterance. Therefore, the middle second might be a section of voice signal that suggested that the utterance was more or less severe than it was. This happened only in one case in the study in Chapter 5, but the example illustrates the problem in using the middle 1-second section.

It would seem that, if the middle portion of a vowel does not appear to be representative of the entire utterance, then additional measurements should be made. One suggestion may be that a number of samples from different points along the signal could be analysed and a mean value taken. The number of samples (and at what intervals) that are required to produce a representative mean is a subject for further research.

Vowel versus connected speech analysis

A further methodological issue is the relationship between the analysis of a portion of a prolonged vowel and the overall voice quality of the patient. A patient may produce considerably different voice qualities between the two separate tasks of producing a prolonged vowel sound and speaking (Karnell et al., 1991). In the situation in which acoustic measurement of the vowel utterance is not a representative measure of dysphonic severity, a different measurement procedure may be necessary (Dejonckere, 1984; Hurme and Sonninen, 1986; Kitzing, 1986; Lofqvist, 1986). Takahashi and Koike (1975) stated that the initial and final parts of voicing may carry abundant information not contained in the steady-state vowel. Similarly, Hammarberg et al. (1980) stated that 'changes in running speech such as vocal onset and termination, voice breaks, etc., are important to voice quality, and are not likely to appear in a single vowel sound' (page 441).

Long time average spectra (LTAS) is one technique that provides information about the spectral distribution of the speech signal over a period of time (Kitzing, 1986; Kitzing and Ackerlund, 1993). The speech signal represents the product of the laryngeal source and the vocal tract resonance. The latter differs for different sound segments but, if the data undergo an averaging process (i.e. as in the LTAS process), the short-term variations caused by phonetic structure will be averaged out and the resulting values will be more representative of aspects of the sound source. However, techniques for acoustically analysing connected speech have some major problems. There are a number of speech/articulatory variables that may contaminate the acoustic analysis. For example, within a connected speech sample, the noise component of voiceless consonants, the speech pauses and the articulatory characteristics of the speaker (e.g. habitual sibilant /s/) may severely distort the data (Sundberg, 1986). These problems have meant that most authors have preferred to analyse prolonged vowel utterances in isolation despite the problems therein (Hillenbrand et al., 1994; Wolfe et al., 1995).

It is likely that there will be many new developments in the acoustic analysis of connected speech, to make it the more preferred option in the future. If continuous speech data are to be used for acoustic analysis, a minimum duration of speech material is required to stabilise long-term measurement of perturbation (Laver et al., 1992). Hiller et al. (1984) found that a 40-second sample was needed in order to provide sufficient data to calculate reliably stable long-term acoustic parameters for healthy male and female speakers. It is unknown how long a speech sample would need to be for a given dysphonic patient.

It would appear that acoustic analysis techniques require further development before they can be used as robust measures of voice change. For example, the reliability of acoustic analysis of dysphonic voices has not received much attention in the literature.

Karnell et al. (1991) compared the acoustic voice perturbation measures of three different analysis systems and they found significant variations in jitter and shimmer measurements across systems. They did not, however, report on the internal variations found within each system. Fitch (1990) studied the test–re-test reliability of perturbation measures on 112 normal vowel utterances, and found that the measures differed significantly. Fitch concluded that perturbation measures should be interpreted with caution and that studies should quote reliability data as well as reporting clinical findings. Studies that have used acoustic analysis to measure longitudinal voice change have not presented data on test–re-test reliability of the technique.

Another major problem in the application of acoustic analysis techniques to measure vocal change is the large inter-subject variability (Kitajima, 1981; Zyski et al., 1984; Kasuya et al., 1986), and the subsequent overlap between normal and pathological populations. This latter point has been the major problem in establishing acoustic analysis as a means of screening for voice pathology in the general population (Von Leden and Koike, 1970; Kitajima et al., 1975; Murray and Doherty 1980; Zyski et al., 1984; Kasuya et al., 1986; Laver et al., 1986). Zyski et al. (1984) analysed a variety of acoustic parameters in a group of 72 subjects (20 normals, 52 pathological cases). The results demonstrated that between 21% and 77% of the pathological cases were included within the range of the normal subjects. Laver et al. (1986) and Banci et al. (1986) also showed a considerable overlap between the acoustic values of pathological and normal voices, which resulted in a number of 'false-positive' findings in their screening programmes. Kasuya et al. (1986) found an overall error score of 25% when analysing the acoustic signal for 'normalised noise energy' in 250 voice samples (including 64 normal controls). In some pathological subgroups, the error score was even higher (e.g. laryngitis = 50%).

Despite these problems of variability, several studies have successfully used acoustic analysis to demonstrate differences between treatment groups. Fex et al. (1994) presented the raw data on six acoustic measures (before and after therapy) for the ten patients in their study.

There was a significant difference between acoustic values before and after, measured on all patients for pitch perturbation quotient (PPQ) and amplitude perturbation quotient (APQ), but not the other four acoustic parameters (two types of normalised noise energy, fundamental frequency and level differences). The PPQ and APQ values appear to be very similar for all patients in the study (although no measures of central tendency or dispersion are quoted). The values for the other four acoustic parameters appear to be more varied and this may explain why they were not shown to be statistically significant in indicating change in the patients in the study.

Roy and Leeper (1991) showed the considerable amount of variance within the 17 patients in the study. However, the size of the change from pre-treat to post-treat for the shimmer and S/N ratio values meant that a significant result was still recorded. There was not a significant difference between the pre- and post-treatment jitter values.

Examination of the acoustic analysis in Chapter 5 shows that the median and range of S/N ratio, jitter and shimmer scores differ considerably from subject to subject. The extent of the range of acoustic measures is, of course, partly the result of the inherent variability between people. However, there are many other factors that may, at least in part, explain the wide range of acoustic values, including:

1. The variety of perceptual dysphonic types (Eskenazi et al., 1990; Wolfe et al., 1991; Hillenbrand and Houde, 1996).
2. The number of different causes for the dysphonia (Beck, 1988).
3. The range of different ages of the subjects (Ramig and Ringuel, 1993; Linville, 1996; Morsomme et al., 1997).

Comparison of acoustic values across subjects is therefore of limited use. The techniques are most profitably used to show relative changes within individual patients. If each patient acts as his or her own control, the difference between the pre- and post-treatment scores can be used to measure voice change.

For acoustic analysis to fulfil its potential as a valuable instrumental measurement of voice and voice change, the techniques require considerable research and development. This development may include work on the reliability, validity, resolution and specificity of acoustic analysis techniques.

Conclusions

Voice is a complex, multi-dimensional phenomenon. Voice therapy requires many complementary skills to effect beneficial change. The therapeutic process is a complex interaction between patient and clinician. The benefits of treatment can be measured in a number of ways. This situation results in an area rich with potential for further research. The purpose of this book is to facilitate understanding of the principles behind effectiveness research. In doing so, the book has highlighted the complexity of this area of study. It was intended as an inspiration for clinicians to become active in clinical effectiveness research – not to daunt people into avoiding it. We should remember that, compared with many areas of medical and paramedical intervention, we are further down the line than we think. We are mature enough as a profession to be critically introspective, and to want to address the needs of the profession over the coming years. In this way, we ensure a continuing improvement in the treatment that we provide to our patients with voice disorders.

References

Abberton E, Fourcin A, Howard DM (1989) Laryngographic assessment of normal voice; a tutorial. Clinical Linguistics and Phonetics 3: 281–96.

Ackerlund L (1993) Averages of sound pressure levels and mean fundamental frequencies of speech in relation to phonetograms: comparison of nonorganic dysphonia patients before and after therapy. Acta Otolaryngologica (Stockholm) 113: 102–8.

Aharony L, Strasser S (1993) Patient satisfaction: what we know about and what we still need to explore. Medical Care Review 50:149–79.

Ah-See KW, Molony NC, Maran AG (1997) Trends in randomized controlled trials in ENT: a 30 year review. Journal of Laryngology and Otology 111(7): 611–13.

Airainer R, Klingholz F (1993) Quantitative evaluation of phonetograms in the case of functional dysphonia. Journal of Voice 7: 136–41.

Altman DG, Bland JM (1996) Absence of evidence is not evidence of absence. Australian Veterinary Journal 74 (4): 311.

Andrews K (1991) The limitations of randomised controlled trials in rehabilitation literature. Clinical Rehabilitation 5: 5–8.

Andrews ML, Schmidt CP (1995) Congruence in personality between clinician and client: relationship to ratings of voice treatment. Journal of Voice 3: 261–9.

Andrews S, Warner J, Stewart R (1986) EMG biofeedback and relaxation in the treatment of hyperfunctional dysphonia. British Journal of Disorders of Communication 21: 353–69.

Arends N, Povel DJ, Os E, Speth L (1990) Predicting voice quality of deaf speakers on the basis of certain glottal characteristics. Journal of Speech and Hearing Research 33: 116–22.

Aronson AE (1985) Clinical Voice Disorders, 2nd edn. New York: Thième.

Bain B, Dollaghan C (1991) Treatment efficacy: the notion of clinically significant change. Language, Speech and Hearing Services in Schools 22: 264–70.

Baken RJ (1987) Clinical Measurement of Speech and Voice. Boston, MA: College-Hill Press.

Banci G, Monin S, Falascci A, De Sario N (1986) Vocal fold disorder evaluation by digital speech analysis. Journal of Phonetics 14: 495–9.

Bassich C, Ludlow C (1986) The use of perceptual methods by new clinicians for assessing voice quality. Journal of Speech and Hearing Disorders 51: 125–33.

Bassiouny S (1998) Efficacy of the accent method of voice therapy. Folia Phoniatrica et Logopaedica 50: 146–64.

Beck JM (1988) Organic variation and voice quality. PhD Thesis, University of Edinburgh.

Beckett RL (1969). Pitch perturbation as a function of subjective vocal constriction. Folia Phoniatrica 21: 416–25.

Bergendal-Fex B (1976) Musical talent testing used as a prognostic instrument in voice treatment. Folia Phoniatrica 28: 8–16.

Black N (1996) Why we need observational studies to evaluate the effectiveness of health care. British Medical Journal 312: 1215–18.

Bless DM (1991) Measurement of vocal function. Otolaryngological Clinics of North America 24 (5): 1023–33.

Bless DM, Hirano M, Feder RJ (1987) Videostroboscopic evaluation of the larynx. Ear, Nose and Throat Journal 66: 363–8.

Bloch CS, Gould WJ, Hirano M (1981) Effect of voice therapy on contact granuloma of the vocal fold. Annals of Otology, Rhinology and Laryngology 90: 48–52.

Blood GW (1994) Efficacy of a computer-assisted voice treatment protocol. American Journal of Speech-Language Pathology 3: 57–66.

Boone D (1982) The Boone Voice Programme for Adults. Oregon: CC Publications.

Boone D (1983) Voice and Voice Therapy, 3rd edn. London: Prentice -Hall.

Boone D, McFarlane SC (1988) The Voice and Voice Therapy, 4th edn. Englewood Cliffs, NJ: Prentice-Hall.

Boston BO (1994) Destiny is in the data. ASHA November: 35–8.

Bough ID, Heur RJ, Sataloff RT, Hills JR, Cater JR (1996) Intrasubject variability of objective voice measures. Journal of Voice 10: 166–74.

Bowling A (1991) Measuring Health. Milton Keynes: Open University Press.

Bradley JV (1968) Distribution-Free Statistical Tests. Englewood Cliffs, NJ: Prentice-Hall.

Brewer DW, McCall G (1974) Visible laryngeal changes during voice therapy. Annals of Otology, Rhinology and Laryngology 83: 423–7.

Bridger MW, Epstein R (1983) Functional voice disorders: a review of 109 patients. Journal of Laryngology and Otology 97: 1145–8.

Brumfitt S (1986) Counselling. Oxon: Winslow Press.

Butcher P, Elias A (1983) Cognitive–behaviour therapy with dysphonic patients: an exploratory investigation. Bulletin of College of Speech Therapists 377: 1–3.

Butcher P, Elias A, Raven R, Yeatman Y, Littlejohns D (1987) Psychogenic voice disorder unresponsive to speech therapy: psychological characteristics and cognitive–behaviour therapy. British Journal of Disorders of Communication 22: 93–109.

Campbell T (1995) Functional treatment outcomes for young children with communication disorders. Presentation to the Academy of Neurogenic Communication Disorders and Sciences. Orlando, FL.

Carding PN (1996) Measuring the effectiveness of voice therapy for patients with non-organic dysphonia. Unpublished doctoral thesis, University of Newcastle upon Tyne.

Carding PN, Horsley IA (1992) An evaluation study of voice therapy in non-organic dysphonia. European Journal of Disorders of Communication 27: 137–58.

Carding PN, Horsley IA, Docherty GJ (1999) A study of the effectiveness of voice therapy in the treatment of forty-five patients with non-organic dysphonia. Journal of Voice 13(1): 76–113.

Carlson E (1995) Electrolaryngography in the assessment and treatment of incomplete mutation in adults. European Journal of Disorders of Communication 30: 140–9.

Casper JK, Colton RH, Brewer DW (1985) Selected therapy techniques and laryngeal physiology changes in patients with vocal fold immobility. In: Lawrence V, ed. Transcripts of the 14th Symposium: Care of the Professional Voice, Part II. New York: The Voice Foundation.

Cochrane AL (1972) Effectiveness and Efficiency: Random Reflections on Health Services. London: Nuffield Provincial Hospital Trust.

Coleman RF (1971) Effect of waveform changes on roughness perception. Folia Phoniatrica 23: 314–22.

Coleman RF (1993) Sources of variation in phonetograms. Journal of Voice 7(1): 1–14.

Collins (1991) The Complete Dictionary Oxford: Clarendon Press.

Combs AW, Avila DL, Purkey WW (1971) Helping Relationships Boston, MA: Allyn & Bacon.

Conture E, Wolk L (1990) Stuttering. Seminars in Speech and Language 11: 200–11.

Cooper M (1973) Modern Techniques in Vocal Rehabilitation. Springfield, IL: Charles C. Thomas.

Cooper M (1974) Spectrographic analysis of fundamental frequency and hoarseness before and after vocal rehabilitation. Journal of Speech and Hearing Disorders 39(3): 286–97.

Cox M, Krecicka M (1990) Acoustic evaluation of laryngeal pathology. Folia Phoniatrica 42: 170–3.

Crane SL, Cooper EB (1983) Speech and Language clinician personality variables and clinical effectiveness. Journal of Speech and Hearing Disorders 48: 140–5.

D'Antonio L, Chiat D, Lotz W, Netsell R (1987) Perceptual-physiologic approach to evaluation and treatment of dypshonia. Annals of Otology, Rhinology and Laryngology 96: 187–90.

Darley F, Aronson A, Brown J (1969) Differential diagnostic patterns in dysarthria. Journal of Speech and Hearing Research 12: 246–69.

Davis SB (1977) Acoustic characteristics of normal and pathological voice. In: Speech and Language: Advances in Basic Research and Practice, Chapter 1. California: Academic Press.

Deal RE, Belcher RA (1990) Reliability of children's ratings of vocal roughness. Language, Speech and Hearing Services in Schools 21: 66–71.

Deal RE, Emanuel FW (1978) Some waveform and spectral features of vowel roughness. Journal of Speech and Hearing Research 21: 250–64.

De Bodt M, Wuyts FL, Van de Heyning PH, Croux C (1997) Test-retest study of the GRBAS scale: influence of experience and professional background on perceptual rating of voice quality. Journal of Voice 11(1): 74–81.

Dejonckere PH (1984) Comparison between long-time-average-spectra of the voice and the sonographic degree of hoarseness according to Yanagihara's classification. International Journal of Rehabilitation Research 7(1): 73–4.

Dejonckere PH, Obbems C, de Moor GM, Wienke GH (1993) Perceptual evaluation of dysphonia: reliability and relevance. Folia Phoniatrica 45: 76–83.

Demming WI (1982) Out of the Crisis. Boston, MA: Cambridge Press.

Diaz JM, Gress CD, Hillman RE (1991a) Using PC-AUDED: Audio editor and analysis programme for the study of periodic segments. Boston, MA: Massachusetts Eye and Ear Infirmary, Voice and Speech Laboratory.

Diaz JM, Gress CD, Hillman RE (1991b) Using PC-AUDED utilities: Average, Filter and Segan. Boston, MA: Massachusetts Eye and Ear Infirmary, Voice and Speech Laboratory.

Dikkers FG, Schutte HK (1991) Benign lesions of the vocal folds: uniformity in assessment of clinical diagnosis. Clinical Otolaryngology 16: 8–11.

Dixon S, Booth A, Perrett K (1997) The application of evidence-based priority setting in a District Health Authority. Journal of Public Health Medicine 19(3): 307–12.

Drudge MK, Phillips BJ (1976) Shaping behaviour in voice therapy. Journal of Speech and Hearing Disorders 49: 398–411.

Dunnet CP, MacKenzie K, Sellars GC, Robinson K, Wilson JA (1997) Voice therapy for dysphonia – still more art than science? European Journal of Disorders of Communication 32: 333–43.

Ellwood P (1988) Shattuck Lecture – Outcome management: technology of patient experience. New England Journal of Medicine 318: 1549–56.

Emanuel FW, Lively MA, McCoy JF (1973) Spectral noise level and roughness rating for vowels produced by males and females. Folia Phoniatrica 25: 110–20.

Enderby P (1992) Outcome measures in speech therapy; impairment, disability, handicap and distress. Health Trends 24: 61–3.

Enderby P, Emmerson R (1995) Does Speech and Language Therapy Work? A Review of the Literature. London: Whurr Publishers.

Eskenazi L, Childers DG, Hicks DM (1990) Acoustic correlates of vocal quality. Journal of Speech and Hearing Research 33: 298–306.

Fabre P (1957) Un procede lectrique d'inscription de l'accoulement glottique au cours de la phonation. Bulletin of Natural Medicine 141: 66–99.

Fairbanks G (1960) Voice and Articulation Drillbook. New York: Harper & Row.

Fallowfield L (1995) Questionnaire design. Archives of Disease in Childhood 72: 76–9.

Fant GH (1960) Acoustic Theory of Speech Production. The Hague: Mouton.

Fant GH (1986) Voice acoustics and dysphonia. Journal of Phonetics 14: 345–7.

Faure MA, Muller A (1989) Stroboscopy. Journal of Voice 2: 15–27.

Fawcus M (1986) Voice Disorders and Their Management. London: Croom Helm.

Fex B, Fex S, Shiromoto O, Hirano M (1994) Acoustic analysis of functional dysphonia: before and after voice therapy (accent method) Journal of Voice 2: 163–7.

Fineberg HV (1990) The quest for causality in health services research. In: Sechrest E, Perrin E, Bumker J, eds. Conference Proceedings: Strengthening Causal Interpretation of Non-experimental Data. Rockville, MD: US Department of Health and Human Services.

Finlay PM, Dawson F, Roberston AG, Soutar DS (1992) An evaluation of functional outcome after surgery and radiotherapy for intra-oral cancer. British Journal of Oral and Maxillofacial Surgery 30: 14–17.

Fisher HB, Logemann JA (1970) Objective evaluation of therapy for vocal nodules: a case report. Journal of Speech and Hearing Disorders 35: 277–85.

Fitch JL (1990) Consistency of fundamental frequency and perturbation in repeated phonations of sustained vowels, reading and connected speech. Journal of Speech and Hearing Disorders 55: 360–3.

FitzGibbon CT (1986) In defence of randomised control trials, with suggestions about the possible use of meta-analysis. British Journal of Disorders of Communication 21: 117–124.

Fourcin AJ (1974) Laryngographic examination of vocal fold vibration. In: Wyke B, ed. Ventilatory and Phonatory Control Systems. Oxford: Oxford University Press, pp

315–33.

Fourcin AJ (1981) Laryngographic assessment of phonatory function. In: Ludlow CL, Hart MO, eds. Proceedings of the Conference on the Assessment of Vocal Pathology. ASHA Reports 11: 116–27.

Fourcin A, Abberton E, Miller D, Howells D (1995) Laryngograph: speech pattern element tools for therapy, training and assessment. European Journal of Disorders of Communication 30: 101–16.

Frattali CM (1998) Measuring Outcomes in the Speech–Language Pathology. New York: Thième.

Freeman M (1986) Management of the dysphonic patient. In Fawcus M, ed. Voice Disorders and their Management, Chapter 6. London: Croom-Helm.

Fritzell B (1986) Voice acoustics and dysphonia. Journal of Phonetics 14: 345–7.

Fritzell B, Hammarberg B, Gauffin J, Karisson I, Sundberg J (1986) Breathiness and insufficient vocal fold closure. Journal of Phonetics 14: 549–53.

Froeschels E (1952) Chewing method as therapy. Archives of Otolaryngology 56: 427–34.

Gerratt BR, Kreiman J (1993) The utility of acoustic measures of voice quality. In: Wong D, ed. Workshop on Acoustic Voice Analysis: Proceedings. Iowa City, IA: National Center for Voice and Speech.

Gladman JRF (1991) Some solutions to problems of the randomised controlled trial in rehabilitation research. Clinical Rehabilitation 5: 9–13.

Gordon M (1986) Assessment of the dysphonic patient. In: Fawcus M, ed. Voice Disorders and their Management, Chapter 2. London: Croom-Helm.

Gould WJ, Korovin GS (1994) Laboratory advances for voice measurements. Journal of Voice 8: 8–17.

Gramming P (1988) The phonetogram: an experimental and clinical study. Dissertation, Lund University, Malmö, Sweden.

Gramming P, Gauffin J, Sundberg J (1986) An attempt to improve the clinical usefulness of phonetograms. Journal of Phonetics 14: 421–7.

Gramming P, Sundberg J, Ackerlund L (1991) Variability of phonetograms. Folia Phoniatrica 43: 79–92.

Greene M (1980) The Voice and Its Disorders, 4th edn. Tunbridge Wells: Pitman Medical.

Greene M, Mathieson L (1989) The Voice and Its Disorders, 5th edn. London: Whurr Publishers

Gupta PC, Witty J, Wright N (1993) An approach to consumer feedback in an outpatient specialty service. International Journal of Health Care Quality Assurance 6: 513–16.

Hacki T (1996) Comparative speaking, shouting and singing voice range profile measurement: physiological and pathological aspects. Logopedics, Phoniatrics and Vocology 21(3–4): 123–31.

Hammarberg B, Fritzell B, Gauffin J, Sundberg J (1986) Acoustic and perceptual analysis of vocal dysfunction. Journal of Phonetics 14: 533–47.

Hammarberg B, Fritzell B, Sundberg J, Wedin L (1980) Perceptual and acoustic correlates of abnormal voice qualities. Acta Otolaryngologica 90: 441–51.

Hartmann E, Cramon D (1984) Acoustic measurement of voice quality in central dysphonia. Journal of Communication Disorders 17: 425–40.

Havas T, Priestley J (1993) The revised Australian fibrescope profile. Journal of Voice 7(4): 377–82.

Haynes WO, Oratio AR (1978) A study of client's perceptions of therapeutic effectiveness. Journal of Speech and Hearing Disorders 43: 21–33.

Hayward A, Simmons R (1982) Relaxation groups with dysphonic patients. Bulletin of the College of Speech Therapists 359: 1–3.

Hecker MHL, Kreul EJ (1971) Descriptions of the speech of patients with cancer of the vocal folds. Part 1; measures of fundamental frequency. Journal of the Acoustical Society of America 49: 1275–82.

Hillenbrand J (1987) A methodological study of perturbation and additive noise in synthetically generated voice signals (1987) Journal of Speech and Hearing Research 30: 448–61.

Hillenbrand J, Houde RA (1996) Acoustic correlates of breathy vocal quality: dysphonic voices and continuous speech. Journal of Speech, Language and Hearing Research 39(2): 311–22.

Hillenbrand J, Biggam DF, Wilde MD (1984) AVR: a computer program for the measurement of perturbation and signal-to-noise ratio in sustained vowels. Evanston, IL: Northwestern University [computer program].

Hillenbrand J, Cleveland, R, Erikson R (1994) Perturbations in vocal pitch. Journal of Speech and Hearing Research 37: 769–78.

Hiller S, Laver J, MacKenzie J (1984) Durational aspects of long term measurements of fundamental frequency perturbations in connected speech. Edinburgh University of Linguistics. Work in progress 17: 59–76.

Hillman RE, Delassus Gress C, Hargrave J, Walsh M, Bunting G (1990) The efficacy of speech and language pathology intervention: voice disorders. Seminars in Speech and Language 11: 297–309.

Hillman RE, Holmberg EB, Perkell JS, Walsh M, Vaughan C (1989) Objective assessment of vocal hyperfunction: an experimental framework and initial results. Journal of Speech and Hearing Research 32: 373–92.

Hirano M (1981) Clinical Examination of Voice. New York: Springer-Verlag.

Hirano M (1989) Objective evaluation of the human voice; clinical aspects. Folia Phoniatrica 41: 89–144.

Hirano M, Bless DM (1993) Videostroboscopic Examination of the Larynx. London: Whurr Publishers.

Hirano M, Hartmann HG (1986) Aspects of videostroboscopy in practice. Proceedings of 20th IALP Congress, Tokyo Press, pp 402–7.

Hirano M, Hibi S, Terasawa R, Fujiu M (1986) Relationship between aerodynamic, vibratory, acoustic and psychoacoustic correlates in dysphonia. Journal of Phonetics 14: 445–56.

Hiraoka N, Kitazoe Y, Ueta H, Tanaka S, Tanabe M (1984) Harmonic intensity analysis of normal and hoarse voices. Journal of the Acoustical Society of America 76: 1648–51.

Holbrook A, Rolnick MJ, Bailey CW (1974) Treatment of vocal abuse disorders using a vocal intensity controller. Journal of Speech and Hearing Disorders 39: 298–303.

Hollien H, Jackson B (1973) Normative data on the speaking fundamental characteristics of young adult males. Journal of Phonetics 1: 117–20.

Hollien H, Paul P (1969) A second evaluation of the speaking fundamental frequency characteristics of post-adolescent girls. Language and Speech 12: 119–24.

Holm C (1971) L'évolution de la phonation de la première enfance a la puberté: un étude électroglottographique. Journal Français d'Oto-Rhino-Laryngologie 20: 437–40.

Hope T (1995) Evidence based medicine and ethics. Journal of Medical Ethics 21: 259–60.

Horii Y (1975) Some statistical characteristics of voice fundamental frequency. Journal of Speech and Hearing Research 18: 192–201.

Horii Y (1979) Fundamental frequency perturbation observed in sustained phonation. Journal of Speech and Hearing Research 22: 5–19.

Horii Y (1980) Vocal shimmer in sustained phonations. Journal of Speech and Hearing Research 23: 202–9.

Horsley I (1982) Hypnosis and self-hypnosis in the treatment of psychogenic dysphonia: a case report. American Journal of Clinical Hypnosis 24: 277–83.

Howard D (1986) Beyond randomised controlled trials; the case for effective case studies of the effects of treatment in aphasia. British Journal of Disorders of Communication 21: 89-l03.

Huff D (1954) How to Lie with Statistics. New York: WW Norton & Co.

Hurme P, Sonninen A (1986) Acoustic, perceptual and clinical studies of normal and dysphonic voice. Journal of Phonetics 14: 489–92.

Iezoni LI (1994) Risk Adjustment for Measuring Health Care Outcomes. Ann Arbor, MI: Health Administration Press.

Imaizumi S. (1986) Acoustic measures of roughness in pathological voice. Journal of Phonetics 14: 457–62.

Jacobsen E (1934) You Must Relax. New York: McGraw.

Jacobson BH, Bush C (1996) Voice Handicap Index and clinician's perceptual judgements; a comparison. Paper presented at the ASHA Convention, Seattle, Washington.

Jacobson BH, Johnson A, Grywalski C Silbergleit A, Jacobson G, Benninger MS, Newman CW (1999) The Voice Handicap Index: development and validation. American Journal of Speech and Language Pathology in press.

Jenkinson C, Coulter A, Wright L (1993) Short form 36 health service questionnaire. British Medical Journal 306: 1437–40.

Johnson IM, Carding PN, Heywood SI, Relf G (1996) A system for measuring the larynx endoscopically. Clinical Otolaryngology 21(4): 34–8.

Johnson TS (1983) The efficacy of treatment; voice disorders. In: Perkins WH, ed. Communication Disorders: Voice. New York: Thième-Stratton.

Johnson TS (1985) VARP – Voice Abuse Reduction Programme. New York: Taylor & Francis.

Kane M, Wellen CJ (1985) Acoustical measurements and clinical judgements of voice quality in children with vocal nodules. Folia Phoniatrica 37: 53–7.

Karnell MP, Hall KD, Landahl KL (1995) Comparison of fundamental frequency and perturbation measurements among three analysis systems. Journal of Voice 9(4): 383–93.

Karnell MP, Scheree RS, Fischer LB (1991) Comparison of acoustic voice perturbation measures among three independent voice laboratories. Journal of Speech and Hearing Research 34: 781–90.

Kasuya H, Masubuchi K, Ebihara S, Yoshida H (1986) Preliminary results on voice screening. Journal of Phonetics 14: 463–8.

Kay NJ (1982) Vocal nodules in children – aetiology and management. Journal of Laryngology and Otology 96: 731–6.

Kent RD (1993) Vocal tract acoustics. Journal of Voice 7(2): 97–117.

Kilman AW (1981) Vibratory pattern of the vocal folds. Folia Phoniatrica 33: 73–99.

Kim KM, Kakita Y and Hirano M (1982). Sound spectrographic analysis of the voice of patients with recurrent laryngeal paralysis. Folia Phoniatrica 34: 123–33.

Kitajama K (1981) Quantitative evaluation of the noise levels in pathological voice. Folia Phoniatrica 33: 115–24.

Kitajima K, Tanabe M, Isshiki N (1975) Pitch perturbation in normal and pathological voice. Studia Phoniatrica 7: 17–23.

Kitzing P (1985) Stroboscopy, a pertinent laryngological examination. Otolaryngology 14: 151–75.

Kitzing P (1986) LTAS criteria pertinent to the measurement of voice quality. Journal of Phonetics 14: 477–482.

Kitzing P, Ackerlund L (1993) Long-term average spectrograms of dysphonic voices before and after therapy. Folia Phoniatrica 45: 53–61.

Klatt DH, Klatt LC (1990) Analysis, synthesis and perception of voice quality variations amongst male and female listeners. Journal of the Acoustical Society of America 87: 820–57.

Klich RJ (1982) Relationships of vowel characteristics to listener ratings of breathiness. Journal of Speech and Hearing Research 25: 574–80.

Klingholz F (1987) The measurement of signal to noise ratio in connected speech. Speech Communication 6: 15–26.

Kluppel-Vetter D (1985) Evaluation of clinical intervention: accountability. Seminars in Speech and Language 6: 55–65.

Koike Y (1973) Application of some acoustic measures for the evaluation of laryngeal dysfunction. Studia Phonologica 7: 17–23.

Kojima H, Gould WJ, Lambiase A (1979) A computer analysis of hoarseness. Journal of Acoustical Society of America 18: 19–49.

Komiyama S, Watanabe H, Ryu S (1984) Phonographic relationships between pitch and intensity of the human voice. Folia Phoniatrica 36: 1–7.

Kotby MN, Abul-Ela MY, Orabi AA (1995) Voice range profiles as a quantitative measure of vocal function: normative data. In: Kotby MN, ed. Proceedings of The World Congress of the IALP, Cairo, 6–10 August, 1995: pp 46–9.

Kotby MN, El-Sady SR, Basiouny SE, Abou-Rass, YA, Hegazi MA (1991) Efficacy of the accent method of voice therapy. Journal of Voice 5(4): 316–20.

Koufman JA, Blalock PD (1982) Classification and approach to patients with functional disorders. Annals of Otology, Rhinology and Laryngology 91: 372–7.

Koufman JA, Blalock PD (1991) Functional voice disorders. Otolaryngological Clinics of North America 24:5 1059–73.

Kratochwill TR, Levin JR (1994) Single-case Research Design and Analysis. New Jersey: Lawrence Erlbaum Associates.

Kreiman J, Gerrat BR, Precoda K (1990) Listener experience and perception of voice quality. Journal of Speech and Hearing Research 33: 103–15.

Kreiman J, Gerratt BR, Kempster GB, Erman A, Berke GS (1993) Perceptual evaluation of voice quality: review, tutorial, a framework for future research. Journal of Speech and Hearing Research 36: 21–40.

de Krom G (1993) A Cepstrum-based technique for determining a harmonics to noise ratio in speech signals. Journal of Speech and Hearing Research 36: 254–66.

de Krom G (1994) Consistency and reliability of voice quality ratings for different types of speech fragments. Journal of Speech and Hearing Research 37: 985–1000.

Lancer JM, Syder D, Jones AS, Le Boutillier A (1988) The outcome of different management patterns for vocal cord nodules. Journal of Laryngology and Otology 102: 423–7.

Laver J, Hillier S, Mackenzie-Beck J (1992) Acoustic waveform perturbations and voice disorders. Journal of Voice 2: 115–26.

Laver J, Hiller S, Mackenzie J, Rooney E (1986) An acoustic screening procedure for the detection of laryngeal pathology. Journal of Phonetics 14: 517–24.

Laver J, Wirz S, MacKenzie J, Hiller S (1981) A perceptual protocol for the analysis of vocal profiles. Work in Progress 14: 139–55.

Leach C (1979) Introduction to Statistics. Chichester: Wiley & Sons.

Lecluse FL, Brocaar MP, Verschurre J (1975) The electroglottograph and its relation to glottal activity. Folia Phoniatrica 27: 215–44.

Liberman P (1961) Perturbations in vocal pitch. Journal of the acoustical Society of America 33: 597–603.

Light RJ, Pillemer DB (1984) Summing Up: The Science of Reviewing Research. Boston, MA: Harvard University Press.

Linville SE (1996) The sound of senescence. Journal of Voice 2 (1):190–200.

Llewellyn-Thomas HA, Sutherland HJ, Hogg SA, Ciampi A, Harwood AR, Keane TJ et al. (1984) Linear analogue self-assessment of voice quality in laryngeal cancer. Journal of Chronic Diseases 37: 917–24.

Lofqvist A (1986) The long-time-average spectrum as a tool in voice research. Journal of Phonetics 14: 471–5.

Ludlow C (1981) Research needs for the assessment of phonatory function. ASHA Reports 11: 3–8.

MacCurtain F, Fourcin A (1982) Applications of the electro-laryngograph waveform display. In: Lawrence Van L, ed. Transcripts of the Tenth Symposium of the Care of the Professional Voice, Part II. New York: The Voice Foundation, pp 51–7.

McDowell I, Newell C (1987) Measuring Health: A Guide to Rating Scales and Questionnaires. Oxford: Oxford University Press.

McFarlane SC, Watterson TL (1991) Clinical use of Laryngograph and the electroglottogram with voice disordered patients. Seminars in Speech and Language 12(2): 108–14.

McGlashan JA, de Cunha D, Harris T, Fawcus R (1995) A system for 3D surface reconstruction of the vocal folds. In: Proceedings of the 23rd World Congress of the Association of Logopaedics and Phoniatrics, Cairo.

McIntyre J (1981) Therapy for a straight forward case of mechanical dysphonia. Bulletin of College of Speech Therapists 351: 2–4.

Martin S (1987) Working with Dysphonics. Oxon: Winslow Press.

Martin S, Darnley L (1992) The Voice Sourcebook. Oxon: Winslow Press.

Maxwell RJ (1992) Dimensions of quality revisited: from thought to action. Quality Health Care 1: 171–7.

Michel JF (1968) Fundamental frequency investigation of vocal fry and harshness. Journal of Speech and Hearing Research 11: 590–4.

Milne R, Hicks N (1996) Evidence-based purchasing. Evidence Based Medicine 1(4): 101–2.

Moncur JP, Brackett IP (1974) Modifying Vocal Behaviour. New York: Harper & Row.

Montague JC, Hollien H (1978) Perceived voice quality disorders in Down's syndrome children. Journal of Communication Disorders 6: 76–87.

Moore A, McQuay H, Gray JAM (eds) (1995) Evidence-based everything. Bandolier 1(12): 1.

Morris RJ, Brown WS Jr (1996) Comparison of various automatic methods for measuring mean fundamental frequency. Journal of Voice 10: 159–65.

Morrison M, Rammage L (1994) The Management of Voice Disorders. London: Chapman & Hall Medical.

Morsomme D, Jamart J, Boucquey D, Remacle M (1997) Presbyphonia: voice differences between the sexes in the elderly. Comparison by phonation time, phonation quotient and spectral analysis. Logopedics, Phoniatrics and Vocology 22 (1): 9–15.

Motta G, Cesari U, Iengo M, Motta JR (1990) Clinical application of electroglottography. Folia Phoniatrica 42: 111–17.

Mueller PB, Larson GW (1992) Voice therapy practices and techniques: a survey of voice clinicians. Journal of Communication Disorders 25: 251–60.

Mulrow CD (1994) Rationale for systematic reviews. British Medical Journal 309: 597–9.

Mulrow CD, Oxman AD (eds) (1997) Glossary: Cochrane Collaboration Handbook. In: The Cochrane Library [database on disk and CDROM]. The Cochrane Collaboration. Update Software, issue 4.

Murray T, Doherty ET (1980) Selected acoustic parameters of pathological and normal speakers. Journal of Speech and Hearing Research 23: 361–9.

Murty GE, Carding PN, Lancaster P (1990) An outpatient system for glottographic measurement of vocal fold vibration. British Journal of Disorders of Communication 26: 115–23.

Mysak D (1959) Pitch and duration characteristics of older males. Journal of Speech and Hearing Research 2: 46–54.

Neiboer GL, De Graaf T, Schutte HK (1988) Esophageal voice quality judgement by means of the semantic differential. Journal of Phonetics 16: 417–37.

Norton R (1983) Communicator Style. Beverley Hills, CA: Sage.

Olsen BD (1972) Comparisons of sequential interaction patterns in the therapy of experienced and inexperienced clinicians in the parameters of articulation, delayed language, prosody and voice disorders. Unpublished Doctoral dissertation, University of Denver.

Olswang LB (1993) Treatment efficacy research: a paradigm for investigating clinical practice and theory. Journal of Fluency Disorders 18: 125–131.

Olswang LB (1998) Treatment efficacy research. Chapter 6 in Frattali CM Measuring Outcomes in the Speech-Language Pathology. New York: Thième.

Pemberton C, Priestley J, Russell A, Havas T, Hooper J, Clark P (1993) Characteristics of normal larynges under flexible fibrescope and stroboscopic examination. Journal of Voice 7(4): 382–90.

Perkins WH (1981) Preventing functional dysphonia. ASHA Convention. Los Angeles, CA: Centre for Study of Communication Disorders.

Perkins WH (1985) Assessment and treatment of voice disorders: state of the art. In: Costello, D, ed. Speech Disorders in Adults, Chapter 4. Windsor: NFER-Nelson.

Prater RJ, Swift RW (1984) Manual of Voice Therapy. Boston, MA: College-Hill.

Prosek RA, Montgomery AA, Walden BE, Hawkins DB (1987) An evaluation of residue features as correlates of voice disorders. Journal of Communication Disorders 20: 166–8.

Prosek RA, Montgomery AA, Walden BE, Schwartz DM (1978) EMG biofeedback in the treatment of hyperfunctional disorders. Journal of Speech and Hearing Disorders 43: 282–94.

Rabinov CR, Kreiman J, Gerrat BR, Bielamonwicz S (1996) Comparing reliability of perceptual and acoustic measures of voice. Journal of Speech and Hearing Research 40: 233–4.

Ramig RL, Ringuel RL (1993) Effects of physiological ageing on selected acoustic characteristics of voice. Journal of Speech and Hearing Research 26: 22–30.

Ramig LO, Verdolini K (1998) Treatment efficacy: voice disorders. Journal of Speech, Language and Hearing Disorders 41: S101–16.

Ranford HJ (1982) Casebook: 'Larynx – NAD'. Bulletin of the College of Speech Therapists 359: 5.

Rao PR, Blosser J, Huffman NP (1998) Measuring consumer satisfaction. In: Frattali CM, ed. Measuring Outcome in Speech-Language Pathology, Chapter 4. New York: Thième.

Reed VW (1982) The electroglottograph in voice teaching. In: Lawrence VL, ed. Transcripts of the Tenth Symposium in the Care of the Professional Voice. New York: The Voice Foundation.

Rogers C (1981) Client-Centred Therapy. London: Constable.

Rontal E, Rontal M, Rolnick M (1975) Objective evaluation of vocal pathology using voice spectrography. Annals of Otolaryngology 84: 662–71.

Rosenfeld, RM (1995) Reading between the lines in medical journals. New Orleans, LA: AAO-HNS Instruction Program.

Roy N, Leeper HA (1991) Effects of the manual laryngeal musculoskeletal tension reduction technique as a treatment for functional voice disorders: perceptual and acoustic measures. Journal of Voice 7: 242–9.

Sackett DL, Rosenberg WM, Gray JAM, Haynes RB, Richardson WS (1995) Evidence based medicine: what it is and what it isn't. British Medical Journal 312: 71–2.

Sataloff RT (1991) Professional Voice: The Science and Art of Clinical Care., New York: Raven Press.

Saxman JH, Burk KW (1967) Speaking fundamental frequency characteristics in middle-aged females. Folia Phoniatrica 19: 167–72.

Schiavetti N, Sacco PR, Metz DE, Silter RW (1983) Direct magnitude estimation and interval scaling of stuttering severity. Journal of Speech and Hearing Research 26: 568–73.

Schmidt CP (1989) Individual differences in perception of applied music teaching feedback. Psychology of Music 17: 110–22.

Schmidt CP, Andrews ML (1993) Consistency in clinician's and client's behaviour in voice therapy: an exploratory study. Journal of Voice 7: 354–8.

Schneider P (1993) Tracking change in dysphonia: a case study. Journal of Voice 2: 179–88.

Shearer WM (1972) Diagnosis and treatment of voice disorders in school children. Journal of Speech and Hearing Disorders 37: 215–21.

Shipp T, Izdebski K (1975) Vocal frequency and vertical larynx positioning by singers and nonsingers. Journal of the Acoustic Society of America 58: 1104–6.

Silverman FH (1977) in Research Design in Speech Pathology and Audiology. Englewood Cliffs, NJ: Prentice-Hall.

Sorensen D (1992) Communicator style characteristics of speech-language pathology students. ASHA 34: 67–70.

Sorenson D, Horii Y, Leonard R (1980) Effects of topical anaesthesia on voice fundamental frequency perturbation. Journal of Speech and Hearing Research 23: 274–83.

Stell PM, ed. (1987) Scott-Brown's Otolaryngology. London: Butterworths.

Stemple JC (1984) Clinical Voice Pathology. New York: Macmillan.

Stemple JC (1993) Voice research: so what? A clearer view of voice production, 25 years of progress; the speaking voice. Journal of Voice 7: 293–300.

Stemple JC, Lee L, D'Amico B, Pickup B (1994) Efficacy of vocal function exercises as a method of improving voice production. Journal of Voice 8: 271–8.

Stemple JC, Weiler E, Whitehead W, Komray R (1980) Electromyographic biofeedback training with patients exhibiting a hyperfunctional voice disorder. Laryngoscope 90: 471–6.

Stephenson J, Imrie J (1998) Why do we need randomised controlled trials to assess behavioural interventions? British Medical Journal 316: 611–13.

Stoicheff ML (1981) Speaking fundamental frequency characteristics of non-smoking female adults. Journal of Speech and Hearing Research 24: 437–41.

Stone RE, Sharf DJ (1973) Vocal changes associated with the use of atypical pitch and intensity levels. Folia Phoniatrica 25: 91–103.

Strandberg TE, Griffith J, Hollowell MW (1971) A case study of psychogenic hoarseness. Journal of Speech and Hearing Disorders 36: 281–6.

Streiner DL, Norman CR (1989) Health Measurement Scales: A Practical Guide to Their Development and Use. Oxford: Oxford University Press.

Sundberg J (1986) Voice acoustics and dysphonia. Journal of Phonetics 14: 345–7.

Takahashi H, Koike Y (1975) Perceptual dimensions and acoustic correlates of pathological voices. Acta Otolaryngologica Supplementum 338: 3–24.

Titze IR (1990) Interpretation of the electroglottographic signal. Journal of Voice 4(1): 1–9.

Titze IR (1994) Towards standards in acoustic analysis of voice. Journal of Voice 8(1): 1–7.

Toohill RJ (1975) The psychosomatic aspects of children with vocal nodules. Archives of Oto-laryngology 101: 591–5.

Van Thal JH (1961) Dysphonia. Speech Pathology and Therapy 4: 1.

Verdolini-Marston K, Burke MK, Lessac A, Glaze L, Caldwell E (1995) Preliminary study of two methods of treatment for laryngeal nodules. Journal of Voice 9(1): 74–85.

Von Leden H, Koike Y (1970) Detection of laryngeal disease by computer technique. Archives of Otolaryngology 91: 3–10.

Ware JE (1993) Measuring patient's views: optimum outcome measures. British Medical Journal 306: 1429–30.

Wedin S, Ogren JE (1982) Analysis of the fundamental frequency of the voice and its distribution before and after voice training. Folia Phoniatrica 34: 143–9.

Weismer G, Liss J (1991) Reductionism is a dead end in speech research. In: Moore C, ed. Dysarthria and Apraxia of Speech. Baltimore, MA: Brookes, pp 15–27.

Welch AR (1982) The practical and economic value of flexible system laryngoscopy. Journal of Laryngology and Otology 96: 1125–9.

Wendahl RW (1966a) Some parameters of auditory roughness. Folia Phoniatrica 18: 26–32.

Wendahl RW (1966b) Laryngeal analog synthesis of jitter and shimmer. Folia Phoniatrica 18: 98–108.

Wendler J (1992). Stroboscopy. Journal of Voice 6: 149–54.

Wendler J, Doherty ET and Hollien H (1980). Voice classification by means of long-term speech spectra. Folia Phoniatrica 32: 51–60.

Wertz RT (1993) Efficacy of various methods. In: Paradis M, ed. Foundations of Aphasia Rehabilitation. London: Croom Helm.

Wilson DK (1987) Voice Problems in Children, 3rd edn. Baltimore, MD: Williams & Wilkins.

Wilson JA, Dreary IJ, Scott S, Mackenzie K (1995) Functional dysphonia (editorial) . British Medical Journal 311: 1039–40.

Wolfe V, Cornell R, Fitch J (1995) Sentence/vowel correlation in the evaluation of dysphonia. Journal of Voice 3: 297–303.

Wolfe V, Cornell R, Palmer C (1991) Acoustic correlates of pathological voice types. Journal of Speech and Hearing Research 34: 509–16.

Wolfe V, Fitch J, Cornell R (1995) Acoustic prediction of severity in commonly occurring voice problems. Journal of Speech and Hearing Research 38: 273–9.

Wolfe V, Steinfatt TM (1987). Prediction of vocal severity types within and across voice types. Journal of Speech and Hearing Research. 30: 230–40.

Wolpe J (1973) The Practice of Behaviour Therapy, 2nd edn. New York: Pergamon Press.

World Health Organization (1980) International Classification of Impairments, Disabilities, Handicaps: A Manual for Classification Relating to the Consequences of Disease. Geneva, Switzerland: WHO.

Yamaguchi H, Yotsukura Y, Sata H, Wantanabe Y, Hirose H, Kobayahi N, Bless DB (1993) Pushing exercise programme to correct glottal incompetence. Journal of Voice 7: 250–6.

Yanagihara N (1967a) Hoarseness: investigation of the physiological mechanisms. Annals of Otorhinolaryngology 76: 472–88.

Yanagihara N (1967b) Significance of harmonic changes and noise components in hoarseness. Journal of Speech and Hearing Research 10: 531–41.

Yeaton W, Sechrest L (1981) Critical dimensions in the choice and maintenance of successful treatments: strength, integrity and effectiveness. Journal of Consulting and Clinical Psychology 49(2): 156–67.

Yumoto E, Gould W, Baer T (1982) Harmonics to noise ratio as an index of the degree of hoarseness. Journal of Acoustical Society of America 16: 1544–50.

Yumoto E, Sasaki Y, Okamura H (1984) Harmonics to noise ratio and psychophysical measurement of the degree of hoarseness. Journal of Speech and Hearing Research 27: 2–6.

Zailouk A (1963) The tactile approach to voice placement. Folia Phoniatrica 15: 147–51.

Zwitman DH, Calcaterra TC (1973) The silent cough method for vocal hyperfunction. Journal of Speech and Hearing Disorders 38: 119–25.

Zyski BJ, Bull GL, McDonald WE, Johns ME (1984) Perturbation analysis of normal and pathologic larynges. Folia Phoniatrica 36: 190–8.

Subject Index

Author index